Posture Power

Posture Power

How to move well, and why it matters

Eleanor Dalton

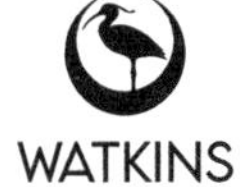

WATKINS

Posture Power
Eleanor Dalton (Posture Ellie)

First published in the UK and USA in 2026 by Watkins,
an imprint of Watkins Media Limited, Unit 11, Shepperton House,
83–89 Shepperton Road, London N1 3DF

enquiries@watkinspublishing.com

Editorial Director: Ella Chappell
Commissioning Editor: Sophie Blackman
Editorial Assistant: Caitlin Nolan
Typeset by Lapiz
Illustrator: Glen Wilkins
Head of Design: Karen Smith
Production: Uzma Taj

Typeset in Minon Variable Concept & Haboro Serif
Printed and bound by CPI Group (UK) Ltd, Croydon, CR0 4YY

The manufacturer's authorised representative in the EU for product safety is: eucomply OÜ – Pärnu mnt 139b-14, 11317 Tallinn, Estonia, hello@eucompliancepartner.com, www.eucompliancepartner.com

A CIP record for this book is available from the British Library

ISBN: 978-1-83681-004-9 (Hardback)
ISBN: 978-1-83681-005-6 (eBook)

10 9 8 7 6 5 4 3 2 1

www.watkinspublishing.com

This book is dedicated to every single client of mine: past, present and future. You have each taught me so much about how the human body and mind work, and you have allowed me to make my passion my career. Thanks for putting your trust in me with the most precious thing you have.

Before we get started, I'd like to state that this book truthfully represents my experience, research and thoughts as they are right now. Some of the things I write, and think, will change over time, as my knowledge deepens and my experience grows. Despite being nearly a decade into this work, I am constantly surprised by the new concepts and ideas that continue to transform my understanding and teaching.

I am truly grateful to you for picking up this book. I hope that you learn something new and that I help you understand how you can incite change from within and take charge of your life.

Moving humans are powerful humans.

CONTENTS

PART ONE
INTRODUCTION TO POSTURE

CHAPTER ONE
HUMANS IN CAPTIVITY

Why are so many of us living in physical and mental angst?

It seems to me that we are no longer human beings; we are human endings, often limping toward the finish line.

The modern world is significantly different from the one we evolved to live in. Because our world is working almost entirely against our primal human nature, many of us – aside from the ever-shrinking hunter-gatherer communities in small pockets of the world* – are merely surviving rather than thriving.

Once upon a time, not so long ago, humans had to move to survive, largely in the pursuit of food. Nowadays, we are often only motivated to move because we feel the need to work off the food we have eaten. This upside-down situation is problematic for our health. As humans, we are programmed to conserve energy, and this makes sense within the context of the limited resources found in the environment we evolved to live in. In a nutshell, humans want to chill out as much as they can: always have, always will. However, life before the First Agricultural Revolution (c12,000 BC, pages 46–7)[1] did not

* When anthropologists study and hypothesize the realities of the day to day lives of our hunter-gatherer ancestors, they look at evidence such as excavated bones and artefacts to piece things together. However, in this book, I mainly use data taken from the study of modern-day hunter-gatherer groups across the world, as we all lived their type of lifestyle until a few hundred generations ago.

Not so long ago, humans had to move to survive, largely in the pursuit of food.

allow us the luxury of relaxing. Despite our innate desire to conserve energy, we were forced to move to find food and shelter – to exist.

In our modern world, most of us are only active by choice. Can you see the problem here? If we are programmed to conserve energy, choosing to move is not going to be particularly high on our agenda. We are wired to seek convenience and quick hacks, and – to our credit – this desire has led to some of the greatest innovations in history.

Throughout this book, it may seem like I am dismissing the wonders of our technological advancements, or that I am romanticizing the hunter-gatherer lifestyle; I'm not. I am looking at things purely from a logical perspective and demonstrating what our bodies have evolved for and what we are doing with them today. This is to help you understand that our lives today are not at all "normal" when we compare them with those of our ancestors. Looking at common modern-day ailments and afflictions from a historical perspective offers more insight and guidance, I think, than viewing things solely through the lens of medical science.

Modern innovations of convenience, which started many thousands of years ago with the invention of tools like the plough, are negatively impacting the function of our bodies and minds. Now that we have well and truly left behind the active outdoors lifestyle of the hunter-gatherer, we suffer at the hands of, what I label, diseases of behaviour and environment. These diseases are ones that many of us accept as a normal part of life: joint and muscle aches and pains, heart disease, Type 2 diabetes, osteoarthritis, osteoporosis, allergies, asthma and so much more.[2]

These ailments have not been statistically significant in present-day hunter-gatherer communities,[3] but they are becoming increasingly more so as these communities are further impacted by modernization. This suggests that many things we consider to be genetic, or an inevitability of the ageing process, are actually symptoms of the long-term impact of our "captivity". I believe it is helpful to think of our modern lives as being the human equivalent of living in a zoo. We are those anxious pacing animals you see penned in their enclosures, who simply cannot thrive because they have been removed from their homeland and the environment they are designed for.

I say, enough! We must actively choose to create a life less convenient for ourselves if we do not want to be debilitated by our lifestyle in the future. Admittedly, this requires going out of our way to make difficult choices and to fight against our primal desire to conserve energy, but this type of lifestyle will get us feeling our best in the long term.

In this book, I want to help you step back into life as a thriving human being. One way you can do this is by leaning into your primal needs through natural movement and play, rather than pretending you can outsmart them with technology. Often, this technology is marketed as a "solution" to our sedentary lifestyle. But the standing desk keeps us still, stuck inside and glued to our screens, and we use the smartwatch to tell us when we have done "enough" steps, rather than sensing intuitively if our body feels tired or restless and in need of more activity.

I am aware that there are many things we can change to give our bodies what they need: improving diet and sleep quality; reducing stress; using fewer chemical cleaning products; reducing artificial light exposure and spending more time outdoors, to name but a few. In *Posture Power*, I highlight how important moving *well* is for our health and wellbeing. This is the area I can help you with.

Posture exercises can be adapted and modified to suit almost any body. While the most important prerequisite is your willingness and ability to commit, long term, to integrating a posture practice into your lifestyle (I recommend three 30-minute sessions per week initially, increasing to almost daily sessions once you've caught the bug), the only limiting factor is your ability to sense and communicate pain levels. If you have the mental capacity to assess whether the exercises exacerbate your levels of pain or tension (and so stop those that do), you are able to benefit from posture therapy.

In terms of equipment, posture exercises are very accessible and can usually be done with objects you already have at home. Depending on pain and mobility levels, exercises can be done from a chair, from a standing position or even from a bed. I have helped all manner of people, including those who are bed-bound, young children with pain, older people who find standing difficult and fairly high level athletes. Children, however, tend to be the most challenging, as they often lack the client accountability and understanding needed. I find it is often better to wait until a child is ready (voluntarily) to make posture exercises part of their lifestyle.

Most of us already know that movement is good for us, but many experts (those whose advice we typically seek for our aches and pains) do not know how to help us learn to move well – at a pace and in a way that the body and nervous system can handle. The cells and tissues in our body have spent a lifetime morphing and adapting away from our hunter-gatherer blueprint, and it will take time to rewire them back to a healthier state.

There are a lot of personal trainers, yoga teachers and other movement professionals out there who help and encourage their clients to move more. However, because often they don't focus on restoring the fundamentals of human movement first, I believe many are innocently leading us toward more pain, tension and fatigue. Excessive movement in a non-human way – in a body riddled with nervous system dysregulation, and muscular and joint imbalance – can do more harm than good.

The problem is that our modern bodies often cannot handle moving more straightaway. The load is too extreme, due to the way in which our body tissues have weakened over time. In order to learn to move well, we must first get the body in balance, to then prepare it for the rigours of moving more. Both stages are important.

When we move well, we can experience a pain-free body and the sheer unadulterated joy that comes from movement. The purpose of this book is to get you started on reclaiming the joy you deserve.

Why me?

I can help you because I am proof that almost anyone can go from having a desk-based job, living in an anxious, stiff and not very healthy body, knowing absolutely nothing about movement, not enjoying exercise at all and absolutely hating science at school, to living and breathing everything about movement – and discovering the life-changing benefits of doing so. Finding joy in movement has given me a new career. I have a burning passion to endlessly learn more, a flexible strong pain-free body and an ever-increasing level-headedness that I didn't think possible for my previously worrisome self. My enthusiasm for how much I have changed my own life with these principles drives me strongly to want to help others.

Although I have several somatic qualifications (posture therapist, yoga teacher, sports massage therapist and breathwork instructor), I don't like to identify with any one of these too much. I am constantly pursuing new avenues to build upon and widen my knowledge, so I can best help my existing clients and, hopefully, you too. Nowadays, I keep it simple and describe myself as a movement teacher because, I teach people how to move better. I show them how to wake up new muscles, improve their posture, relax a heightened nervous system, breathe properly, remedy imbalanced and dysfunctional movement patterns and, importantly, transform how they feel in a physical, mental and spiritual sense. I believe frequent movement is a fundamental part of being a happy, fulfilled and calm person and that too many of us are missing out on the dose we need. This lack of movement impacts so much more than our muscles and joints, as we will explore throughout the book.

I don't believe you need a medical degree to help yourself (or other people) reduce pain in a productive way; you simply need to use common sense, keep an open mind and continue to learn. Don't get me wrong, if you suffer from any form of acute injury, get yourself to a hospital and don't come my way! Modern technology is incredible in the face of an emergency: for example, if you need bones set, a blood transfusion or any other critical surgery. However, I don't think that other types of modern technology, such as long-term reliance on medication and painkillers, or even orthopaedic procedures, are the best response to many chronic diseases or conditions. In fact, I think our reliance on and trust in these types of remedies to "save us" often takes us further away from truly attaining better health. Chronic diseases and conditions often improve when we make simple lifestyle changes to better mirror the life for which we have evolved.

I believe frequent movement is a fundamental part of being a happy, fulfilled and calm person.

The lifestyle changes we need to implement are fairly straightforward and, I believe, should come intuitively to us as humans. I am writing this book not as a scientist or expert quoting complicated statistics and studies, but as a regular person trying to use my experience, intuition and logic to help you. The more we think we require the expertise of other people to help us achieve good health, the more elite, complicated and out of reach achieving good health will seem.

I firmly believe we already have everything it takes to become the healthiest version of ourselves. I want to help you get started with the basics, and then teach you to relearn how to trust your inner knowing. Although I can guide you, everyone is different and you will have to figure out what works and what doesn't for your individual body. This is about taking accountability and stepping into your power. Once you have learned my methods, the real joy lies in the fact that you can do it all yourself, from the comfort of your own home, every day for the rest of your life.

> I firmly believe we already have everything it takes to become the healthiest version of ourselves.

What is my approach?

If you are here because you'd like to reduce your pain or stay pain-free naturally, without any medical interference, I think it's important that I speak authentically from my own experience. That way, I hope I can convince you that your goal is possible. Some of those around me are starting to blame their age for their aching joints and tense muscles. I do not move perfectly, nor do I have perfect posture, but I am extremely active. I have enough muscles in my body that work functionally to keep myself moving reasonably efficiently, and I remain pain-free.

I believe that most of us can improve our movement patterns to the point where we feel significantly different, even if we never become fully pain-free. This is still a positive outcome, and hope and optimism are powerful tools in staying motivated toward recovery and change. I can't and won't teach you how to push your body to the absolute limit to achieve superhuman physical feats. My goal is to help you reduce your pain and improve your day to day life.

To do this, I see the whole human body as a connected unit. As I will explain throughout the book, moving well reduces most types of musculoskeletal pain and many other symptoms you may think are unrelated (such as breathing, digestive, circulatory and neurological issues). Every single part of the human body needs to be exercised and considered when it comes to being pain-free (including often forgotten parts such as the diaphragm, toes, fingers and calves). This is because the whole body is connected through various muscular and fascial chains. Like the "butterfly effect", what happens in one part of your body can have a dramatic effect on another.

To truly get to the root causes of our movement issues, and create meaningful dramatic change for ourselves, we need to understand how all the parts and systems of the body are interconnected. Many of us are stuck in a modern-day cycle of symptom suppression (a general term used to describe ways and means of avoiding feeling pain, explored in chapter 5) and are not addressing the root causes of the pain. This cycle includes things like taking painkillers, having steroid shots, wearing padded shoes, insoles or knee braces, orthopaedic surgery, icing, hot baths and avoiding movement. None of these will resolve why we have pain in the first place and will, in fact, just push the problem to return (and get worse) another day. Hiding signals of pain is not the same as tackling the reason why the pain is there. I am here to help you with the latter.

When we learn how to gently and correctly restore the function back to all the muscles in our body and create more balanced movement patterns to ease aching joints, we also restore so much more within us. Better and more frequent movement results in a better life all round. The physical pain within our body dramatically reduces, the daily anxiety and overwhelm of having to deal with pain lessens, we are more peaceful within our buzzing modern brains and we renew a sense of confidence in our ability to be the masters of our own healing journey. Not only that, but everything else inside the body will work more harmoniously, too. We'll breathe better, suffer less digestive upset and toilet more easily; our central nervous system will deliver messages more efficiently; we'll have better coordination and balance, better blood circulation and lymphatic movement, and we will be clearer headed. By improving our posture, we naturally improve everything that resides inside our posture.

I believe that relearning how to move well is an important key to unlocking the door to an entirely different life. A life that always belonged to you, but that the modern world took away and made you forget. You are in charge. You are powerful. Your body is your lifelong home – look after it.

TEST YOUR POSTURE

Let's start the book with a postural bang. To begin your journey toward unpicking the puzzle that is your body, I'd like you to do a practical posture test. This will kick-start your transformation into becoming a curious 'posture detective' for your own body: someone who is able to interpret the signals their body is sending out.

By picking up this book, you have taken the first step and your life is about to get a whole lot better. But, before it can, you need to take stock of your current postural situation.

See what you find out about yourself by following the Standing at Wall posture test. It will tell you a whole lot about your body.

There are a few more of these posture tests peppered throughout the book.

Can you stand up straight?
Standing at Wall posture test

If asked whether you can stand up straight, your immediate response may well be, "Yes, of course." However, if we were in a room together, my response would probably be, "No, you can't." This is because there is a difference between merely standing and standing well.

All you need to do is to stand with your back against a wall for five minutes, with a few of my postural alignment cues to consider along the way. It's the postural alignment cues that may open your eyes and make you realize that standing up straight perhaps isn't as simple as it looks.

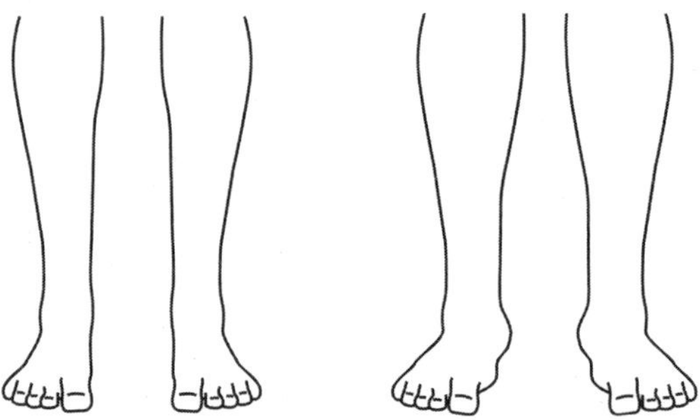

Figure 1: Parallel feet (left) versus out-turned feet (right). Notice how the middle of the second and third toes, rather than the big toe joints, line up with the ankle.

1. Take off your shoes and stand with your back against the wall. Your feet need to be hip-width apart and parallel (fig. 1). Please note that hip-width is narrower than you think and parallel is more pigeon-toed than you think. Imagine car tyre alignment: the centre of your second and third toes need to align with the middle of the front of your ankle, knee and hip. We don't want to use the big toe joint as our measure of parallel foot alignment.

2. Both calves need to be touching the wall.
3. Your bottom needs to be touching the wall.

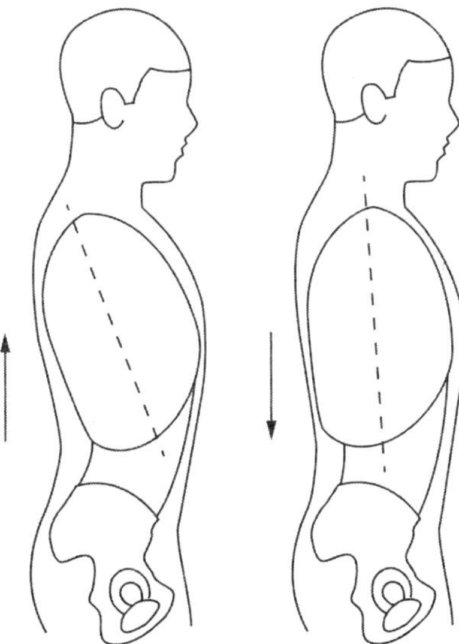

Figure 2: Flared ribcage (left) versus neutral ribcage (right). You'll probably find you want to flare your ribcage upward to bring your shoulders and head back to the wall. I want you to keep your lower ribcage against the wall, even if that makes you feel rounded forward in your shoulders and head.

4. Your lower ribcage needs to be touching the wall (fig. 2). This is critical to standing well and I will explain why after the posture test. This postural alignment cue is the one that your body and brain will most likely struggle with the most.
5. Without changing the angle of your lower ribcage position against the wall, your shoulders, backs of arms and head should be relaxed and touching the wall. Yes, really!
6. Finally, you should be able to relax your belly, hands and jaw and maintain a calm, steady, nasal, diaphragmatic breath. This type of breath means that you are breathing

in and out through your nose and engaging your diaphragm as you breathe. Your diaphragm is a key respiratory muscle that domes horizontally at the bottom of your ribcage like an open umbrella. When you are engaging your diaphragm, your upper belly and lower ribcage will move with your breath. You shouldn't notice your collarbone or shoulders move upward as you breathe. If you do, you are chest breathing and not breathing with your diaphragm.

This posture test seems fairly easy, relaxing and comfortable. After all, you're just standing up straight for a few minutes and that's simple, right?

Hold the position for five minutes – how do you feel? Can you maintain the parallel foot alignment? Are both calves touching the wall in a balanced manner? Does your lower ribcage stay against the wall facing forward, or does it want to lift and face up toward the ceiling? Can you maintain the ribcage position and keep your shoulders/head against the wall? Importantly, are you relaxed and maintaining the nasal diaphragmatic breath?

Don't worry, I know this is harder than it looks and I'm going to explain why.

Maintaining the parallel foot position can be difficult. You may feel your ankles and feet working hard – maybe getting hot, red and veiny, and even cramping. This is because most modern shoes switch off the foot muscles, preventing our feet from moving and properly supporting the other joints upstream. As we will explore in more detail later in the book (page 106–29), most modern shoes are heeled. Often they have only a marginal raised heel, but it makes a huge difference to the body to be constantly trapped in a heeled position at the foot. As our feet stiffen into this posture over time, we turn out our feet to compensate for the stiffness (a form of "cheating"). Simply standing with your feet parallel and flat to the ground can really challenge stiff feet that are used to being constantly held outward in marginally heeled shoes. This position can wake them up in a new way.

Maintaining both calves against the wall can also be hard. Again, because the heels in most shoes constantly pitch our bodies forward on a diagonal from the ankle (fig. 3), it becomes difficult for many of us to hold a 90-degree angle at the ankle. You might find this position super tiring on your calves if they are not used to holding your ankles at a 90-degree angle.

You may notice that one calf, leg or butt cheek wants to swing away from the wall. This probably indicates that you have a wonky pelvis, because the two sides are behaving differently. It's likely that you have more tension through the hip of the leg wanting to pull away from the wall. If you've spotted this, great! You're beginning to gain more awareness of imbalances in your posture when you can notice this type of thing.

You will probably find it incredibly hard to keep the lower ribcage, shoulders and head against the wall at the same time. This is mainly due to tight hips. When we are sat down, our hips are in a range of motion called flexion. Standing up straight, as we are in this posture test, requires our hips to be able to perform a range of motion called extension (fig. 4).

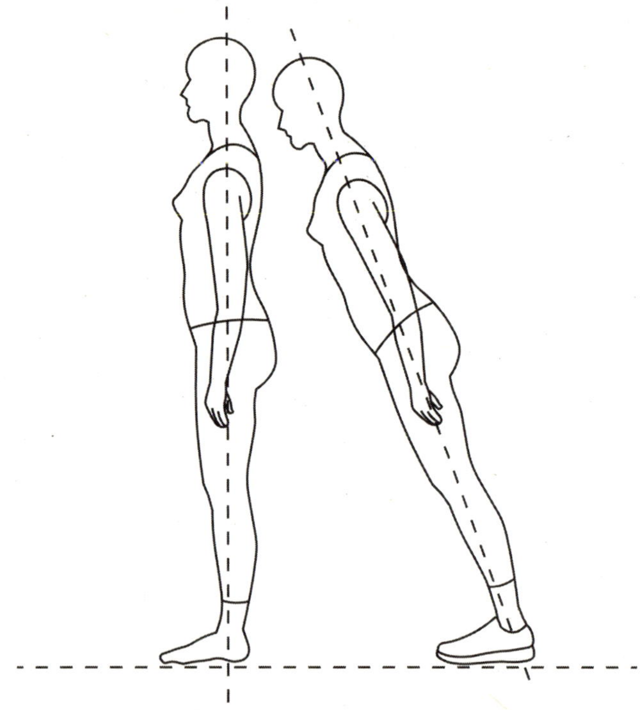

Figure 3: 90-degree angle at the ankle (left) versus pitching forward from the ankle (right). Flat feet keep the joints stacked above each other and supported by the ankle. Even a marginal heel on a shoe pitches the entire body forward, meaning you lose the support you're supposed to get from your ankle.

By the time we are adults, most of us cannot extend our hips functionally – mainly because of the time we spend sitting down passively in a chair in hip flexion. Our body adapts to what we do with it for most of the time. So, if we spend longer in hip flexion than in hip extension, we lose the capacity to extend our hips properly. Our body can, however, trick us (compensate) to make us believe we are achieving hip extension by

Chronic lumbar compression caused by dysfunctional hips is one of the most common causes of lower back pain.

lifting our ribcage up into a flared position and compressing our lower back into hyperextension (an exaggerated curve). This is due to the location of the primary muscles of hip flexion, our iliopsoas muscles (fig. 5).

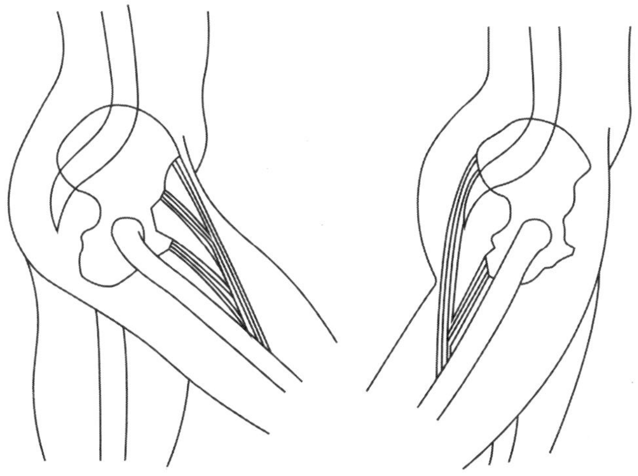

Figure 4: Hip Flexion versus Hip Extension: The closed hip position of flexion when sitting (left) versus the open hip position of extension when standing (right).

Without a good understanding of our posture, many of us have no idea that we are habitually stuck in this flared ribcage and compressed hyperextended lower back posture while we stand, walk, sit or do almost anything. Chronic lumbar compression caused by dysfunctional hips is one of the most common causes of lower back pain, and also many other types of pain around the body.

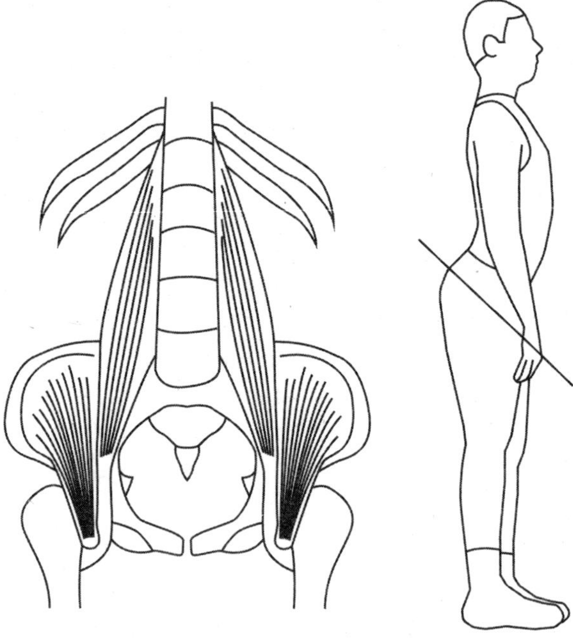

Figure 5: The diagram shows the attachment points of the hip flexors. The primary hip flexors (iliopsoas, left) seizing up can cause a hyperextended lumbar curve (also known as lordosis, right) and a lifted ribcage position.

HOW HIPS AFFECT RIBS

The hip flexor muscles attach around the groin onto the thigh bone (femur), on our pelvic crest, on each lower back (lumbar) vertebra and onto the bottom of the ribcage and diaphragm. The movement and position of the ribcage, therefore, directly impacts how mobile our hip flexors are (and vice versa). When our hip flexors are stiff and cannot extend, this impacts how we stand. Without proper hip extension, the tension pulls between the thigh bone and lower ribcage, and the ribcage flares upward to compensate.

When standing, our brain's postural priority is our head position, because in the past it was important for humans to keep their eyes on the horizon, scanning for danger. Our body subconsciously arranges itself as best it can around this need. By flaring our ribcage, we trick ourselves into feeling like we have upright posture, but we are preventing our lower body and shoulders from moving functionally by doing so.

When we flare our ribcage, the shoulders aren't actually back and the head isn't actually upright. It's an illusion created by the compensation occurring in the lower back on behalf of those pesky tight hips. In the Standing at Wall posture test, when we remove the compensation in the lower back – by keeping the lower ribcage against the wall – we expose the true position of our shoulder girdle and head.

This can come as quite a shock the first time you do it, and you might think you're doing it wrong. If you're surprised by how slumped you feel and how far forward your head, shoulders and arms seem to come, you're doing it right. You're simply feeling exactly what is happening with your posture when you're not compensating with your spine and ribcage.

The key to changing this ribcage flare is to teach your hips to functionally extend. Standing in the posture test position for as long as you can (with the bottom ribs at the wall and slumpy shoulders) can be a great way to improve hip extension. You may notice you become wobbly in your legs – if so, great! This is your hips learning to functionally extend because you're no longer cheating with the ribcage.

If you stand here and tolerate the wobbles for long enough, you may also notice – as if by (posture) magic – that your shoulders and head begin to melt backward effortlessly toward the wall. If this happens, you're experiencing your first glimpse of the butterfly effect within the body. In this example, changing the function of your feet and hips can drastically alter how the upper body is able to hold itself, without doing anything to the upper body at all.

I hope the posture test has got you thinking and perhaps made you a tiny bit more body aware. Hopefully, you're excited to get started.

Before we move on to part 2 and begin to explore what posture is, where most of our posture problems come from and some of the harmful myths that prevent us from truly healing our posture and overall health, I'd like to tell you a little bit more about my story and how I got here.

TAKEAWAYS

1. Our modern environment and lifestyle have warped our sense of what is normal.
2. The human body evolved to lead a hunter-gatherer lifestyle. When it doesn't, it suffers both physically and mentally.
3. We are wired to conserve as much energy as possible, so you are not alone or lazy if you struggle to find the motivation to move.
4. We must actively choose a life less convenient to optimize our health in a suboptimal environment.
5. Moving more intensely, without first restoring muscular function, joint balance and efficient movement patterns, often leads to more aches and pains.
6. If we want to be pain-free and feel our best, we must restore the quality of our movement patterns. This is what I can help you with.
7. The whole body is connected, and we must treat symptoms holistically.

CHAPTER TWO
MY STORY

My symptoms

It's November 2016. Physically I'm sat at my desk in London, but mentally I'm floating above myself watching a weird scene unfold below. I don't quite know what's happening. One moment I am "in my body" experiencing my manager talk to me, feeling like I am disconnected from reality (like I am in a computer game), having to carefully consider my words before I speak and trying hard to make sure I don't come across as weirdly as I feel. The next moment it is like I've zoomed ten feet above my head and am looking down with a bird's-eye view of my hair, desk and manager. Then, I fall back into my body, feeling completely spaced out and terrified at my desk. I am looking at the computer screen, not able to process anything, feeling like I am about to cry – stuck like a caged bird.

Not long after this, my colleague asked me if I was okay, and I burst into floods of tears and was ushered into a private area with my manager. Before I knew it, I was on a train back to the West Midlands (where I am originally from) and was signed off work for two weeks with generalized anxiety disorder. I was never formally diagnosed, but a while later I found out this strange out of body experience is called disassociation and it is a way for the body to cope with stress.

This was one of the most pivotal moments of my life and served as the biggest wakeup call I'd ever have. It sparked much of the dramatic lifestyle change that came for me, and I am – strangely – forever grateful for how desperately unhappy and depressed I was during this period. Without this frightening realization – of how disconnected from myself and my body I'd become, how I wasn't living in the way I wanted, how I was suppressing everything that I should have been feeling and how chronically stressed and mentally unwell I was – I wouldn't have taken the steps to change the trajectory of my life.

Let's rewind the clock a bit. I had a comfortable middle-class childhood, and I got through my teenage years having had a wonderful time at school with amazing friends. As my school years ended, and despite being an fairly high achiever, I had a sense that university wasn't for me. However, I didn't trust myself enough back then to believe in my intuition, so I sort of got funnelled into the university system. This is an early example of me losing faith in my ability to make the right choices for myself.

After university, I was lucky enough to go backpacking with a friend for six months. When I returned, I couldn't face the world of corporate work, so I went to work on a horse farm in Argentina. During this period, the freedom, adventure and outdoors lifestyle helped me reconnect with myself. I felt alive and happy, and it felt right. It was when I got back from Argentina and started working in London that the descent toward my dissociative episodes began.

Despite having a gut feeling that I didn't want to get a "proper" job and move to London, I did. My friends were there, and I felt like it was just what people like me did. I somehow managed nearly five years in the city with a growing sense of malaise as time passed. I was incredibly unhappy. I hated the concrete, the busy environment, the commute, and being sat at a computer all day. I also hated feeling like the money I made and the material things I had dictated my social standing. I hated my life.

At that time, I didn't treat the root cause of my unhappiness. That would have required a great deal of soul searching, taking better care of myself, confronting difficult emotions and implementing monumental change. But I did do a great job of distracting myself by suppressing my symptoms of unhappiness. Rather than changing anything meaningful in my life, I numbed everything out. My partying, drinking, spending and self-sabotage increased, and I felt like every day was a roundabout of unease, insecurity and anxiety. Deep down, I knew I wasn't being myself, but I didn't know what to do about it.

Eventually, after several years of feeling increasingly unhealthy, miserable, negative and cynical, I found myself in 2016. And that's when the panic attacks and disassociation began to happen. I remember coming out of Oxford Circus station one day and feeling like I couldn't breathe. The world was spinning, the noises were crushingly loud, and I felt completely insane. Worryingly, and tellingly, my primary fear was what other people around me would think. These types of events happened a couple of times before the pivotal moment I described at the beginning of the chapter. Each time, I'd get annoyed at my brain for not behaving in the way I wanted. But rather than listening to what my body was trying to tell me (or changing something), I kept pretending it wasn't happening.

Then, of course – because there is only so long you can push things down before something gives – the floating-above-the-desk incident happened, and I got signed off work. This was the circuit breaker I needed. The catalyst for great change.

My resolve

I quit my job, handed in my notice on my rental flat and returned home to live with my mum. I spent a couple of months licking my wounds and feeling pathetic. My memories of that time are ones of feeling crushed and being under a blanket. I no longer had the blood-curdling anxiety, but instead slipped into a sleepy depressive stage for the first time. The daily stresses were in the past, but now I had to confront my absolute lack of purpose, which was even more painful.

For the next few years, I worked in meaningless corporate jobs I didn't like. I was a lot less stressed than I had been in London, but I was a lot more depressed and felt hopeless. Was I really going to spend the next 40 years of my life doing something that sucked away my soul?

During this time, my friend asked me to sign up to run a half-marathon with her. I had never done anything like that before, was completely unfit and a bit overweight. I didn't do any exercise and so was quite scared by the prospect, but I remember thinking, "Why not?" Having the half-marathon to train for gave me something productive and non-work related to focus on. I can't say I enjoyed running particularly, but I did enjoy the mental break it gave me. I felt the health benefits of more movement, and sticking to a healthy habit helped build up my confidence.

Six months later, the half-marathon came and went. It coincided with the start of my third corporate job in the same calendar year. I don't know if it was the improved mindset and confidence that came with the running or just a dawning realization that something needed to change in my life, but I remember telling my mum that this job would be the last one in which I would ever work for someone else. I'd decided I was going to do my own thing, but I didn't yet know what that thing would be.

Despite not having a plan, I knew I'd need money to tide me over. For the first time in my life, I created a daily budget and started saving. I wasn't earning much, but saving became my priority. Whereas, once upon a time, I had seen endless shopping, frequent meals out and impulsive holidays as a necessary escape from my unhappiness, I realized I wouldn't ever get what I wanted if I carried on living this way. Budgeting was another meaningful change I made in my life: it both helped me feel like I was working toward something bigger and made me proud of myself. These little steps were starting to make a real difference in how I thought about myself and what I realized I could achieve with effort and patience.

The next "little" step for me was finding and starting yoga. As the darker nights drew in, I didn't want to run anymore, and for some unknown reason, I had decided that I wanted to become flexible before I was 30. I was almost 28 and, while I didn't suffer any pain, I was as stiff as a board and had a gut feeling that this stiffness was going to come back and bite me in the future. I signed up for a 30-day trial where I got to do as many yoga classes as I wanted. Yoga breathed back into me the life the adult world had sucked out. It was a time of incredible transformation for me: physically, mentally and spiritually.

Yoga breathed back into me the life the adult world had sucked out.

By the end of those 30 days, I was a totally different person. My body was both hardening and softening. Muscles were developing and toning in a way they hadn't before, and my joints were loosening. It was remarkable. I felt so proud of myself for being so committed in that month, and my self-respect grew further. I felt like discovering movement was giving me my life back. Mentally, I hardened and softened, too. I became tougher in my resolve to change my life, but I also became kinder to myself and others around me. For the first time ever, I became interested in spirituality, the bigger questions and the world of "woo-woo". I loved it. I loved the kind people I met through yoga. The ritual of burning incense and sage. The chanting and the mantras. How still and quiet my mind felt, as my body sweated and shook beneath me. I felt like I was coming back to myself each time I stepped on the mat.

My root cause

A year or so after discovering my love for yoga, I began looking for my escape route from the corporate world. I was enjoying my personal adventure into the world of the human body and movement, and I felt passionately about helping other people discover it, too. I considered becoming a yoga teacher but felt my hometown couldn't handle yet another one, so I signed up for a sports massage therapist qualification. Frustratingly, I got to the end of the course only to realize it didn't sit right with me. During the training, we were treating symptoms of pain and tension by massaging out the tight bits. While massage feels pleasant and may lead to some short-term alleviation of muscular tension, it doesn't answer or address why the areas we are massaging are painful or tense in the first place. I finished the course with a question: rather than endlessly massaging out muscular tension, how do we stop muscular tension from forming?

While searching intensely online for an answer to this question, I hit my jackpot: posture therapy. The book *Pain Free* (1998) by Pete Egoscue (I still joke that this is my postural version of the Bible) enlightened me to the fact that tension and pain in the body originate from postural imbalances. And that through corrective exercises, we can create balance throughout the whole body again. By finding this postural balance, we are addressing the root causes of most symptoms of pain and tension and so are truly healing – with no negative side-effects. Finally, I had discovered something I could totally get behind. Something that made utter sense to me and that I believed I could turn into a viable business.

How do we stop muscular tension from forming?

I signed up to train as a posture therapist and soon became a woman obsessed. I spent the next six months practising yoga before work, commuting an hour and a half into work, sitting at my desk all day, commuting back an hour and a half, and then seeing my first "guinea pig" clients in the evenings. I don't quite know how I kept to this schedule, but it was the first time in my life that I felt myself edging closer to liberating myself from the rat race. I had found a fire and purpose within me, and I truly put this down to discovering yoga and then using movement as a mechanism to build upon my new-found self-respect and confidence. The more I moved, the better everything in my life became. It was so simple.

About ten months after reading the posture Bible, I qualified as a posture therapist and left my corporate job. I became "Posture Ellie" full-time, self-employed. I was terrified, but I was free!

Before we dig into posture properly, I'd like to summarize some of the key things I realized while I was going through my painful and lengthy transition, because I believe they apply to every type of true physical and mental transformation. To transform ourselves, we need to differentiate between the symptoms and the root causes of an issue, otherwise we waste time. For me, the symptoms of my issues were unhappiness, anxiety, depression, spending, partying, panic attacks and disassociation, to name but a few. The root causes of my issues were that I had stopped listening to my gut and wasn't living the life that was right for me, and that I had lost my confidence and self-respect along the way.

TAKEAWAYS

1. Symptoms of a problem present differently to the root causes of a problem. Identifying symptoms is more straightforward than admitting to and changing root causes. However, focusing on the symptoms doesn't change the root causes. The more you concentrate on firefighting the symptoms, the longer you'll distract

yourself from fixing the root causes, and the worse both the symptoms and the root causes become.

2. Don't always listen to other people; they don't know what's best for you. No one has all the answers. To grow your confidence and feel aligned with your true self, you need to learn to let your inner compass be your guide.
3. Even if the situation seems hopeless, there is always hope. It takes hard work, mindset shifts and, sometimes, sacrifice. But there is always hope.
4. Regular people, like you and me, can change the trajectory of our life. It's just a question of choosing to make slightly different decisions every day going forward, until we get to where we want to be.

Ultimately, understanding the fundamental difference between focusing on symptoms and tackling root causes is what this book is all about. I believe the reason why so many people are stuck in downward spirals of physical and mental pain is because – in the treatment of chronic musculoskeletal pain – our health system focuses almost exclusively on symptoms. The root causes of our pain nearly always boil down to the fact that we are living modern lives that are entirely out of kilter with our body's primal needs. But the current health system tends to think we can patch over this debilitating mismatch with medication and "band-aid solutions". I say we can't.

So, let's go and learn how to regain our posture power.

PART TWO

POSTURE PROBLEMS AND MYTHS

CHAPTER THREE
PROBLEM NO. 1: DEFINING POSTURE

It's not just about pulling your shoulders back and standing up straight

One of the main issues I face when talking about posture is establishing a universal definition of its meaning. There seems to be a huge chasm between how most of us tend to think of our posture versus how movement therapists like me define posture.*

I have found that many of us consider our posture to be relevant only with regard to how we look while sitting or standing. I often hear things like, "I sit with bad posture," or "My parents always used to tell me off for slouching, so now I pull my shoulders back." This chasm in understanding has also led to some one-dimensional research in which the impact of posture on pain in the body is studied, and no correlation between posture and pain is found.[4] If I were to use these researchers' narrow definition of posture, I would agree with their results. Stiffly holding yourself in a rigid position will not make you feel better than being more relaxed. You might stand tall or sit tall in a chair, but that isn't posture. By my definition, your posture is not about stiffly and artificially holding yourself a certain way.

* This topic is discussed beautifully in episode 173 'Is Posture A Thing?' of the "*Move Your DNA*" podcast by Katy Bowman.

What is posture?

It helps to think of your posture as your movement patterns and your entire musculoskeletal system. Your posture is not one static position; it's a dynamic state of being. It's how your body shows up in the world and how it handles all the activities you do. And, because your posture is about your movement patterns, it's also about the function of your muscles and your nervous system. As we will explore later in the book, posture impacts and involves all the systems in your body, because they all reside inside your posture. Your posture is your house, the vessel your soul lives in, and it is damn important if you want to thrive.

Your posture is not one static position; it's a dynamic state of being.

You do not have a singular posture, but everything you do requires a posture. In my view, your posture really means "the position of your body", and so it is relevant for every movement you perform. You have almost infinite postures. As examples, you have a walking posture, a running posture, a sitting posture and a sleeping posture.

Confusingly, you have the overall posture of your body on a macro level – like the typical "hunched over at a desk" posture that is so synonymous with the word – but you also have posture on a micro level. Sometimes, while you sit at your desk, your hips will be in an internally rotated posture (if you pinch your knees together), but at other times your hips will be in an externally rotated posture (if you have one ankle on the knee of the other leg), for example. You can, on a macro level, be sitting in a "hunched over at a desk" posture but, on a micro level, many different postures can be happening through each joint in your body (e.g. hips, knees, ankles). You, see? It's more complicated than some studies let on.

Your posture – the position of your body in any given movement – reflects to you the quality, efficiency and balance of your movement patterns and how functionally your muscles are working at that time. Is there muscle or joint pain? Is there muscular tension? Are you mobile? Are you stiff? The answers to these questions lie in what your muscles and movement patterns are doing.

So, if we view our posture too simplistically and see it just as pulling back our shoulders and standing up straight, we perpetuate common posture myths. I find myself having to debunk these frequently.

POSTURE MYTHS

Posture myth 1: Our posture has no significance, meaning or impact in relation to our pain levels.
Posture myth 2: Posture is something aesthetic that can be corrected in the moment.
Posture myth 3: There is good or bad posture.

We are going to expand our understanding of the definition of posture by exploring the three posture myths above.

Myth 1: Posture isn't important

If your posture isn't important, it means your muscles aren't important

Unfortunately, the different ways in which society defines posture can severely undermine our understanding of how impactful our posture is to both our short- and long-term physical and mental wellbeing.

As I said previously, your posture is the home you live in. Hair and skin aside, nearly every part of your physical being is housed within your posture, which is dictated by your body's ability to move. Your body's ability to move is dictated by how well your muscles work. And your muscles may not work all that well because, like me, you've lived a life in captivity.

The upright, elegant (yet relaxed) standing posture that we label as "good" is visual information of a body that can easily and naturally hold itself because of its strong muscles and aligned joints. In this position, we are displaying muscular balance from front to back, left to right, inside to outside and top to bottom (fig. 6).

The slouched, depressed-looking, imbalanced standing posture that we label as "bad" is visual information of a body that – due to a lack of whole body muscular strength – cannot hold itself in optimal efficient alignment. This muscular weakness further displays as imbalances across the bones and joints.

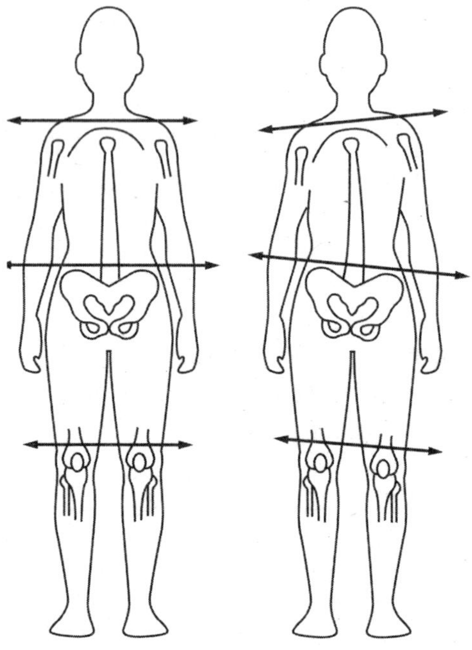

Figure 6: Balanced aligned joints (left) versus imbalanced misaligned joints (right). A balanced body signifies whole body muscular function, whereas an imbalanced body shows muscular dysfunction.

POSTURE PRINCIPLES

The relationship between posture and chronic pain is simple. Our muscles move our bones and hold our bones in place.

1. The phrase "use it or lose it" is key to understanding muscles. Remember, we evolved to conserve as much energy as possible because we lived in an environment where acquiring resources was difficult. Because of this innate survival mechanism, when we do not use certain muscles, our body thinks these parts are unnecessary. It then conserves energy by switching them off.
2. When muscles are underused long term, they fall asleep and stop working properly. We call this "dysfunction", and dysfunctional muscles no longer hold and move the bones efficiently in a biomechanical sense. Bones and joints will become imbalanced because dysfunctional muscles are pulling them out of whack. Imbalanced joints cannot compete with the forces of gravity, and this creates wear and tear in the joints and tension in the muscles. The fewer muscles in your body that work functionally, the stiffer and more stuck your movement patterns will be and the worse you will feel. Other muscles will step in to compensate, but this "overworking" causes exhaustion, which in turn creates tension. Long term, this tension will pull the joints more permanently out of efficient alignment.
3. One of the many fantastic things about the body is that it is incredibly adaptable. So, while the body can conserve energy and switch things off, the reverse is also true. If you begin to demand more of your body, it will be forced to wake up your sleeping muscles. When muscles wake up again and start working properly – that is, become more functional – the increased muscular function holds and

moves the bones more efficiently. The positions of the bones and joints will become more balanced long term.

4. The more muscles in your body that work functionally, the more fluid and mobile your movement patterns will be, and the better you will feel. The more you improve your overall posture, the fewer aches and pains you will have. Balanced joints work synergistically (together) with gravity, and so will not wear away on themselves. Functional muscles will not be overworking and won't need to store tension to keep you upright and move you around.

As you can see, to dismiss posture as unimportant to our health is to basically dismiss our muscles as unimportant to our body. Improving our posture boils down to making sure we maintain the strength and function of our muscles throughout our life.

Over the course of history, human evolution has created an optimal postural blueprint for us. With a small degree of variation, most able-bodied human beings are born with little difference in their bones and physical makeup. While there are different heights and sizes and some structural differences between males and females,* we are pretty much cut from the same cloth.

Unless born with a movement impacting disability, most of us have similar movement capabilities at birth. However, we then go on to have different lives: the way we are raised as children, the traumas and accidents we suffer, the state of our nervous system, our daily habits and activity levels, and our sports and hobbies all create different trajectories

* Differences are partly due to the male and female reproductive systems, but also the physiological demands that come with the tasks of hunting and gathering. Hunting typically fell to the males and gathering to the females, and there are some differences in our structures to allow for this.

for our posture over time. A turbulent childhood that creates a dysfunctional breathing pattern, a sedentary job that leads to tight hips, a lopsided sport like tennis that causes rotation of the spine or a car accident that breaks your pelvis will impact the symbiotic relationship between your muscles, joints and nervous system. Every single thing that ever happens to you bears a mark on your posture.

While we cannot change our life's history, we are, as I said earlier, highly adaptable. We cannot change the car accident that happened to us, but we can retrain our nervous system's response to it: we can relearn how to use our diaphragm, how to unclench our jaw and how to create more balance in our pelvis, lessening the pain. Those of us who can restore, or preferably retain, our posture as close as possible to our predesigned human postural blueprint will lead significantly more comfortable lives.

As we go on to explore through the book, mobile posture equates to less pain, better function of the other systems in the body and more mental clarity and ease.

Myth 2: Stop slouching
Holding yourself rigidly and self-consciously exacerbates the issue

You cannot improve your posture by merely holding yourself a bit differently for a short period of time. Sitting up taller, sucking your belly in or pulling back your shoulders are all, ironically, creating more tension in your body. These common posture corrections that you've probably heard many times are making your posture stiffer, and this in turn will create movement problems and imbalances. Holding yourself rigidly is not natural and not a reflection of how your body really moves. By artificially holding your posture in place, you are feeding the beast you are trying to kill.

There are lots of companies peddling things like posture correctors, cushioned insoles and ergonomic desks. These types of products compound the myth that posture can be corrected in the moment. They trick us into thinking that our posture can be improved by something other than teaching our muscles new or forgotten movement patterns and habits over time. I am here to tell you this is not the case. Your posture can only be changed for the better by learning new movement patterns. This is because learning new movement patterns strengthens and changes our muscles. And as you now know, the state of our muscles dictates our posture.

A posture correcting back brace keeps you locked in a stiff unnatural position. An ergonomic desk allows you to sit still, more comfortably, for hours. The insoles and cushioning in your shoes take the work out of your feet. None of these products strengthen or positively change your muscles. By regularly using these sorts of things, we are subcontracting muscular work that should be happening in our body to external sources of support.

Strong muscles are different to tense muscles. Strong muscles are created through movement and physical challenge, but tense muscles are created by bracing and being still.

You may get some short-term relief by making small changes immediately, but there is nothing you can correct in the present moment to positively impact your real posture, your movement patterns, long term. So, for now, just relax your shoulders and your belly, and let your body be in its natural posture, without rigidity and stiffness.

Myth 3: You can have good or bad posture
All postures are good, but being stuck in one posture is bad

I do not like the words "good" or "bad" in relation to posture.* I prefer to use the terms "stuck" or "mobile" posture, which

* I do sometimes use the terms "good" and "bad" for effect because it helps other people understand postural concepts a bit better.

allow for a lot more nuance and understanding. There is nothing inherently wrong with any position that the human body can perform, and using the word "bad" can demonize completely normal positions and shapes that we want our bodies to be able to make.

Some examples of common supposedly "bad" positions are sitting in a kneeling "W" shape as a child (fig. 7), having your head in front of your shoulders at your desk (fig.8), and having a big arch in your lower back when standing (fig.9). These totally normal human positions only become bad or, as I prefer to say, problematic, when you are stuck in them long term.

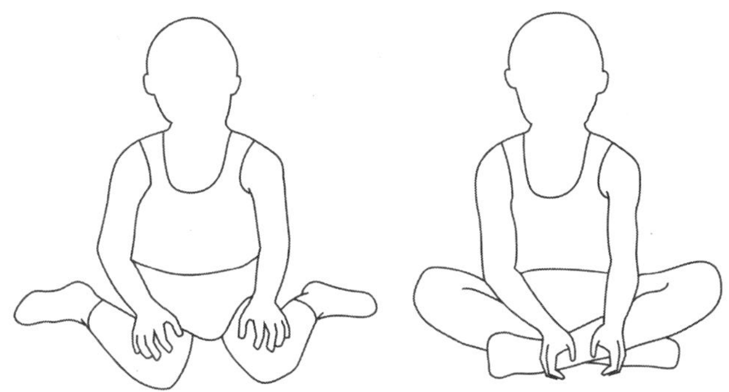

Figure 7: The "W" position, with internal hip rotation (left) versus the cross-legged position, with external hip rotation (right).

A child who spends a long time sitting in internal hip rotation ("W" shape) will need plenty of external hip rotation to balance out their pelvic, femur and knee position. The "W" shape is not bad in itself; it just needs to be counterbalanced regularly to maintain full range of motion at the joints – like any other posture.

A person who spends a lot of time with their head in front of their shoulders at their desk (fig. 8) will also need to spend plenty of time with their head sitting on top of their shoulders or pushing backward into extension to counterbalance the forward flexion. Lying supine in bed without a pillow is a nice way to regularly reset the head position back over the shoulders, as the body lies horizontal and works as a team with the forces of gravity (fig.8).

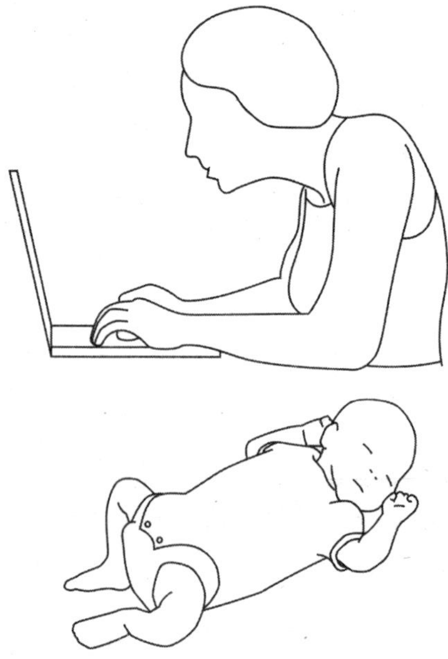

Figure 8: Spinal flexion (above) versus a more neutral spinal position while lying supine (below).

A person whose pelvis is stuck anteriorly in lumbar extension will need to spend time moving their pelvis posteriorly and teaching their lumbar spine to flex to counterbalance the anterior tilt (fig. 9).

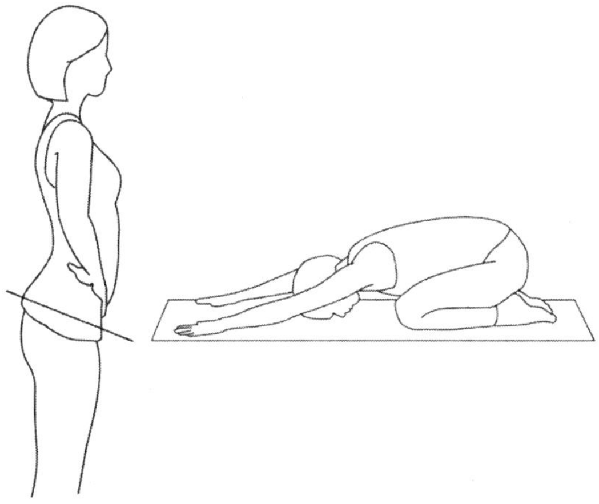

Figure 9: Anterior pelvic tilt (left) versus posterior pelvic tilt (right). An anterior pelvic tilt is a pelvis and lumbar spine in extension. Child's pose puts the pelvis and lumbar spine in flexion (posterior pelvic tilt).

None of the postures mentioned above are bad, but they can be problematic because function and pain are affected when parts of our body become stuck in a particular posture. If our body can easily bring itself out of the supposedly bad position, it's not a problem. But when we spend too long in one posture – without regularly asking our muscles and joints to counterbalance that posture with the opposite range of motion – our muscles get stiff, and this *is* a problem.

When we are stuck in a particular posture, we call this dysfunction. This is because our muscles are no longer able to functionally hold, lever and propel our bones around efficiently. Any area of dysfunction will create a cascade effect throughout the body.

Think of a pebble dropping in water; dysfunction spreads. The gradual degradation of muscular function, caused by our stuck posture, leads to a breakdown in communication between all the muscles and joints. Eventually, this leads to wear and tear in multiple joints and frequent tension in many muscles. As one joint stiffens, it has a ripple effect on the other muscles and joints nearby, and they begin to compensate. Over time, as those nearby joints become exhausted due to overwork, they can no longer cope with the extra burden and they start to become dysfunctional too, spreading the problem onto further joints. And so the parasite of muscular dysfunction spreads throughout the body.

To illustrate this point, using the examples above, the child that spends a lot of time in the internal hip rotation of the "W" shape (without the counterbalancing time spent in external hip rotation) will have hips that eventually become stuck in internal hip rotation. That child will likely, at some point, suffer knee pain from the lack of movement available through their stuck hips. Likewise, the head that becomes stuck in front of the shoulders (and cannot return to a more supported position above the shoulders) will put a perpetual strain through the neck and back. And the arched lumber spine and pelvis that become stuck in extension will eventually put a constant strain on the lower back and prevent the hips from moving functionally, too.

It's not all doom and gloom, though. As I said earlier, the body is incredibly adaptable and the mechanism of "use it or lose it" works both ways. If you start asking your muscles to do new things, they will kick back into action. At any age, you can significantly remedy how stuck you are, by learning new movement patterns, waking up sleeping muscles and rebalancing your joints. This new mobile posture will dramatically reduce the pain previously caused by being stuck, imbalanced and dysfunctional.

Think of posture exercises as being an MOT (a yearly car check to ensure the car is roadworthy) for your body: a regular check-in that lubricates and realigns your joints, and keeps all the moving parts working together safely.

As I hope you are starting to see, mobile posture is extremely important, but it is also extremely simple. If most of the muscles in the body are working properly, we can avoid most types of musculoskeletal pain. However, it only takes a quick look around in the street or a brief listen to your friends and family bemoaning their aches and pains to recognize we have a big problem. Why does almost everyone complain of pain after a certain age? And why do so many of us look hunched forward and move with a degree of imbalance?

I think many of you may already know what the single greatest contributor to our postural decline is. The humble chair.

TAKEAWAYS

1. By posture, I mean your movement patterns. Your posture reflects how well all the muscles in your body are working.
2. Your posture is incredibly important because your muscles are incredibly important.
3. If you want to suffer less musculoskeletal pain and have better function in all the other systems in your body, you need to restore and maintain your muscular function.
4. The only way to improve your posture is by working on the quality, variety and frequency of your movement patterns.
5. You cannot artificially correct yourself or keep yourself still using devices like back braces to improve your posture.
6. Holding yourself stiffly and your joints in unnatural positions is creating more stiffness in your muscles.
7. Using external devices to support your muscles makes the muscles switch off and does not, therefore, improve your posture.
8. There isn't any such thing as good or bad posture, but you can have mobile or stuck posture.

CHAPTER FOUR
PROBLEM NO. 2: THE BIG SLUMP OF HUMANKIND

We're not meant to do the same thing all day long

The root cause of the main movement problem we face is evident. We weren't designed to be strapped in a car seat at birth, to be put in a baby bouncer to contain us as a toddler, to sit still at a desk all day, to go to the toilet in a seated position, to travel by moving chair or to spend so much of our leisure time sinking into a sofa.

Our early ancestors had to move constantly to survive, but today, along with many other evolutionary mismatches that prevent us from achieving optimal health — such as ultra-processed foods and excessive screen time — we simply don't move enough to keep our biology and psychology functioning as they should. How far back this lack of movement goes is hard to say. We have lost sight of what "normal" means (for humanity), because barely anything that we consider normal in our lives is normal in relation to the environment for which our species evolved.

Some of us may already be aware of how much movement has been stripped from our daily activities by technological developments. Studies suggest that the amount of time the average American now spends sitting down each day increased 43 per cent between 1965 and 2009,[5] which means that they are immobile for between 9 and 13 hours of their waking day.[6]

Personally, I didn't have a smartphone until I was 22. And, in my teenage years, surfing the Internet required no one else to be using the landline and a bleepy and slow connecting mechanism. It was an occasional weekly treat. Now, I spend many hours on most days on a smartphone, engaging with the Internet, and this is my new normal. My mother remembers getting her first calculator and having a shared telephone line, but my young niece will never know a world without YouTube or online delivery services. If my niece were to chat to my deceased grandparents, the oldest of whom was born in 1925, about their younger years, she would probably not be able to grasp just how different their lives were as children. If we continue this line of enquiry, we soon get back to a time before motorized transport, electricity and central heating, and I'd like you to think about how these three inventions have changed our movement profiles. Let the changes you can imagine in the past 30 or 300 years help you gain perspective on how much our environment must have altered for our bodies over the past 300,000 years.

As I briefly mentioned earlier, our movement patterns started to change during the First Agricultural Revolution, roughly 12,000 years ago, when humans first began to cultivate crops for food and domesticated animals.[7] This is because with the development of agriculture came more permanent settlements and a move away from the previous hunter-gatherer lifestyle. The more developed we became, the more sedentary we became, as we needed to move less for our survival. Even though 12,000 years is quite an incomprehensible amount of time to conceptualize, it's a drop in the ocean for human history.

The definition of human history is a little murky. You'll find different interpretations depending on which books and studies you read, and how you view the definition of human. When looking at our human timeline, are we only to consider our species, *Homo sapiens*, which emerged around 200,000 to 300,000 years ago?[8] Or do we go back further and consider human history to have started with the oldest proposed species of hominid,* *Sahelanthropus tchadensis*, approximately 6 to 7 million years ago?[9] Or back further when we diverged from gorillas around 9 million years ago? How do we truly decide when human history began, because everything that came before us shaped us as *Homo sapiens*?

Let's go lowball and consider human history to be the past 300,000 years. And let's have a look at where the First Agricultural Revolution sits within it.

In his brilliant book *Primate Change* (2018), Vybarr Cregan-Reid uses a good analogy to help us visualize this. He says that, if we look at our human timeline as a nine to five working day, the First Agricultural Revolution would be at 4.58pm. The Industrial Revolution (approximately mid-18th to late 19th century) would have begun at 4.59pm and 58 seconds. Using this analogy, this means that everything around us – in our modern environment (post-Industrial Revolution) – that we think is normal has only existed for a mere two seconds of human history.[10]

What *is* normal for us?

When we study data gathered from the few remaining hunter-gatherer communities in the world, we find they are active for about six hours a day, on average. They walk between 8 and 16km (5 and 10 miles) a day in the pursuit of food and additionally spend nearly four hours a day engaging in light activity and just over two hours in moderate activity.[11]

Hunter-gatherers spend a lot of time gently moving each day, but they spend a lot of time relaxing, too. Studies show that the Hadza people in Tanzania spend as much as nine hours a day relaxing.[12] However, they are not sitting passively in a chair, leaving the chair to do the work of their muscles.

* All species who more closely appear to be humans rather than chimpanzees or other apes.

Relaxing for hunter-gatherers involves mainly being on the ground in a position that still requires their muscles to work to hold them upright. When they sit on the floor, they only tend to stay still for a maximum of 15 minutes at a time, before moving again.[13] This relaxation time is combined with an active working lifestyle of six hours of movement a day.

These statistics give us some idea as to how much rest and activity our bodies were designed to do each day – just to keep us alive – and it gives us some perspective on where things may be going wrong. Not that long ago (a mere 500 years), it wasn't normal to spend time in any form of chair. Think about how many types of seats you sit in everyday, how many chairs you have at home and how long you spend in them, on average, every day. And imagine how different your body would feel if you never sat in a chair. We have created a new normal.

SITTING STILL

I'd like to caveat that sitting on a chair is not a problem in itself. It is the *amount of time* we spend sitting still, passively, over the course of our lifetime. Any position that we hold for many hours of the day will eventually become problematic for us: standing, squatting, lying down or even balancing on one foot. We are not designed, biomechanically, to do the same few postures over and over every day. The posture itself is not the issue; it is the lack of movement variety. So, in the modern world, sitting becomes a problem because sitting is what most of us do for many hours a day. But, hypothetically, you could input any posture here. It's not the case that "sitting is the new smoking", but, more accurately, "doing the same thing over and over again with little movement variety is the new smoking."

Like many things we consider normal, chairs are a recent invention. We must think of them as a modern technology for which our bodies were not designed, even if that seems strange or confronting. Throughout most of documented history, the people we see in ancient artworks sitting on chairs are gods, royalty or priests. Chairs only became more widely available around the time of the Industrial Revolution,[14] when we developed the technology to mass manufacture more affordable chairs and the newly emerging city-based occupations required more sedentarism. This means that chairs have only been widely used for about 0.055 per cent of the time *Homo sapiens* have been around. In the past 250 or so years, we have gone from spending barely any time to spending 9 to 13 hours each day in some form of chair.

We must ask ourselves, how long would a hunter-gatherer last if they behaved normally (for us) and sat in a chair for this many hours a day? Hunter-gatherers need to move frequently to stay alive, because movement is the ticket to survival when your next meal is not guaranteed. Nowadays, we do not have to think about our survival every moment of the day, but we do need to respect and understand that the hunter-gatherer lifestyle is what the human body is so exquisitely designed for. Our environment may have changed, but our bodies have not. Regardless of when we are born in the grand scheme of human history, our bodies need frequent and varied muscular demand to operate properly and feel at their best.

Supply and demand

As our modern lives don't require enough muscular demand to keep the body healthy, all the muscles across our body weaken. Demand strengthens muscles; lack of demand weakens muscles. When our muscles are not being called upon often enough (and with enough variety), the human body machine stops running efficiently.

I like to picture the human body as a machine full of cogs, levers and connecting parts. Just like a car, as one thing breaks down and loses its function, another part of the machine is impacted and may start to break down, too. For example, if the wear in your car's brake pads is not addressed, it won't be long before your brake discs also wear out.

Your body is the same. Once muscular integrity is lost, the spiral of muscular decay continues until dysfunction (and pain) is present across multiple joints in the body. Our modern lifestyle is damaging our bodies and brains in ways we struggle to see, because we are so deeply entrenched in our version of what is normal. The more normal we think our world and lifestyles are, the more disconnected, disempowered and diseased we become.

So, what is one of the most straightforward routes toward reconnecting to your body and brain, becoming more empowered and intuitive, and experiencing significantly less mental and physical disease?

Improving your posture. And it will change your life.

STANDING STILL

I feel the need to add a sidenote here regarding standing desks, often lauded as the postural saviour for sedentary desk-workers. While standing desks have some advantages over sitting desks – you'll likely fidget more, burn about 8 to 10 per cent more calories[15] and work a few more muscles throughout the day – I do not believe they fix or truly help the problem of sedentarism. Being sedentary is not about sitting; it's about staying still and not challenging the body enough. As I mentioned earlier in this chapter, humans are not designed to remain in one position for lengthy periods. Standing still for many hours a day is no more human than sitting still and passively on a chair for many hours a day – sorry, it's not! Not only that, if you are wearing shoes with even a small raised heel (a typical workplace shoe) or if your standing posture is already imbalanced, standing for a long period of time may exacerbate symptoms of pain and tension throughout your body. There are no real remedies for restoring your posture, other than restoring your movement patterns and moving more.

TAKEAWAYS

1. We spend too much time being still and have been too still for most of our lives.
2. Hunter-gatherers spend about six hours a day moving. They also spend a lot of time relaxing on the floor in different positions that keep them gently working their muscles. They do not traditionally sit in chairs.
3. Even things like chairs must be considered a modern technology for which we haven't evolved.
4. Sitting down itself is not an issue; it is the amount of time we spend sitting down passively in a chair that is the problem.
5. Any static posture in which we are stuck for too long will become problematic.
6. Standing desks are marginally better than sitting desks. No product that keeps us still will truly help our posture. Only improving the quality, variety and frequency of movement will improve our posture.

CHAPTER FIVE
PROBLEM NO. 3: WE SYMPTOM CHASE AND THEN WE SYMPTOM SUPPRESS

We focus on the area that hurts and assume pain is the problem

We all suffer at the hands of the prevailing Western paradigm, which – when it comes to chronic long-term issues – is normally set to symptom chasing and symptom suppression. Let me explain what I mean by these two terms.

First, when we suffer some form of chronic pain or tension, we tend to focus predominantly on the symptom (the area that hurts) and this is called symptom chasing. This behaviour is totally understandable because the symptom may be screaming at us. But just because it's screaming, it doesn't mean it's the actual problem. The location of the symptom is often a red herring, and focusing on the symptom can hugely distract us from finding the root cause of the issue. We will investigate this in greater detail in chapter 7.

Second, once the pain sets in, it doesn't go away – because we haven't got to the root cause of the problem. We then hide from the continuing pain by suppressing our symptoms: taking painkillers, having surgery on the area of pain, stopping activities that cause the pain and pretending the pain

> Pain is a message to be listened to, not ignored.

isn't there. None of these actions addresses the root cause of the pain.

By symptom chasing and symptom suppressing, we are failing to understand the human body as the wonderfully connected, intrinsically linked, fantastically complex, but also beautifully simple movement machine it is. We suffer because of our general misunderstanding of what pain means. Pain is a message to be listened to, not ignored.

The methods I set out in this book will help you get to the root causes of your pain. They will help to heal the symptoms of your pain, so you won't need to suppress them anymore. But before we dig further into this, I will explain why we must listen to pain if we want to be healthy and, ironically, pain-free.

The problem with symptom suppression
Pain is your best friend trying to keep you safe

Pain is a message from the body that something is wrong. It allows us to make changes to bring our body back to safety. Without pain, we would die or suffer serious injury unnecessarily in many scenarios.

For example, if we did not get helpful feedback from our nervous system, we might place and keep our hand on a hot stove while our skin blistered to our bones. Luckily, pain is the friend that tells us to whip our hand away (fig. 10).

In this example of short-term peril, it is obvious that pain is a useful message from our body. However, I believe pain is always a useful message. For this reason, I avoid all manner of "everyday" medication. I find it frightening how easy it is for us to take a pill rather than to respond accordingly to what our bodies are asking for: be that more rest, a better diet, less stress or more exercise. By allowing myself to fully experience my occasional maladies, I am able to read correctly when my body has recovered – and adapt my behaviour and respect the pain until that point.

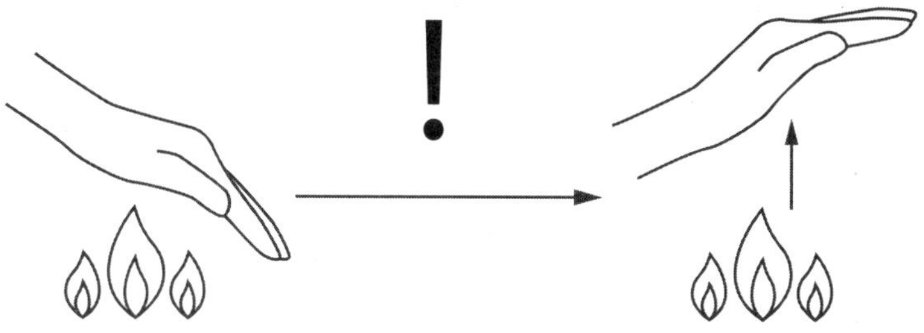

Figure 10: Input + pain message = change of outcome. Pain is a message that is only ever trying to change your behaviour to keep you safe.

In some situations – like having a tooth removed or recovering from surgery – I celebrate the benefits of our ability to numb pain temporarily while something else gets fixed. My issue comes with the long-term use of painkillers or when painkillers are considered a fix in isolation. If we mask our pain, our body continues to suffer under the radar; we're just not receiving the feedback anymore.

Our (understandable) aversion to pain in a quick-fix world is deeply damaging, because it prevents us from establishing the root cause of the problem and truly healing ourselves. For every painkiller we take, every steroid injection we have, every joint that gets scraped of its arthritis, every bursa removal, every vertebra that is fused and every joint replacement that occurs (the pain relief/symptom suppression methods are far reaching – I have not listed them all here), we are temporarily taking away the pain, but we are not addressing the movement problem that is causing the pain. The pain and the movement problem are two different things. By removing the pain, we take away our body's desperate attempts to get us to listen to the warning signs and adapt our behaviour accordingly.

Let's use an analogy to illustrate this point. Imagine you are the monarch of an ancient city, who also rules over a smaller neighbouring village. This village is one of the main suppliers of food for the city. One day, a messenger comes running into your throne room to let you know that another local opposing group has entered the village and ransacked some food from a storage barn. It's already a busy day for you: your children are causing you trouble and there's a big feast happening in the city today. You simply don't have time to deal with this issue, so you send the messenger away. The next day, the messenger returns and tells you the other tribe members are getting more serious. They've now set fire to the barn! Today, you've got to appoint a new courtier and arrange a hunt for next week. You don't have time to deal with the message. To punish the messenger for bothering you again, you throw him in a prison cell overnight. At least that will keep him from interrupting your schedule while you plan the hunt. The next day he is released and sent back to the village. To your huge annoyance, he returns a few days later looking extremely dishevelled. The village has been razed to the ground, most of the villagers are dead, all the food has been plundered, and all the farming equipment has been stolen. This is one interruption too far (you're having your new robes fitted today) and so you decide to execute the messenger.

Finally! Your problem is resolved because the messenger is gone. Well, no. You've got rid of the pain (the messenger), but you haven't addressed the root cause (the raiders). Without the food supply from the village, the city quickly begins to fall into disarray, the people flee for greener pastures and you, the monarch, are left in ruin.

This is what is happening in the body when we "don't have time" to think about our knee/hip/back/foot/shoulder/wrist/*insert any body part here pain and choose a method of symptom suppression instead. We are executing the pain messenger, but we are not dealing with the problem.

This makes it clear we can't outsmart pain. However, when we are suffering pain, often the only solution offered by the medical profession is one of symptom suppression, so what real choice do we have? And, if the professionals don't have any better solutions, what hope is there for us?

This is where the all-important "Posture Paradigm Shift" comes in. (A paradigm shift is a situation in which the usual and accepted way of doing or thinking about something changes completely.)

There is *absolutely* hope for us all, but we need to look at things differently. Symptom chasing prevents us from seeing the bigger picture and makes us lose perspective. Something needs to shift.

The great big Posture Paradigm Shift
Posture therapy sees and treats things differently

Like many movement practices such as yoga or lifting weights, posture therapy teaches us how to wake up weak muscles in our body to better support and move our joints with aligned efficiency. This relieves the stress caused by imbalanced muscles and joints and eases the tension that will eventually lead to wear, tear and pain.

The muscles that need to be woken up will often present in an entirely different part of the body to where you expect. This is because the entire human body is connected through chains of muscles, fascia (connective tissue), tendons, ligaments and bones. When you "pull a string" in one part of the body, the whole "puppet" responds.

In other words, posture therapy doesn't focus on the area of the body that hurts. Instead, it considers how one part of the body may be painful because it's not getting the support it needs from another part elsewhere. For example, if you have a painful back and a disc herniation (slipped or ruptured disc), a posture therapist probably won't advise back stretches or back strengthening exercises and will likely leave your back alone. They will know that the more you meddle with an area of pain, the more likely you are to exacerbate it. Don't poke the bear and all that. Instead, a posture therapist will try and work out why your back is painful and why your discs have slipped out of alignment. This sleuthing involves assessing all the parts of your body and how they move and interact as a whole unit. There is no point looking at your painful back or herniated disc in isolation: no part of the human body works in isolation.

This is the big difference between symptom chasing and discovering the root cause of a problem. Unfortunately, many professionals are currently stuck in a symptom chasing cycle, rather than considering the movement of the body as a connected whole.

> Posture therapy doesn't focus on the area of the body that hurts.

Let's look more deeply. Here's a fictional case study of the current pain paradigm and how a typical symptom chasing and then symptom suppression journey might pan out for someone. Afterwards, I'll explain what I would do differently.

FICTIONAL CASE STUDY:
SYMPTOM CHASING AND SYMPTOM SUPPRESSION

Joanne, aged 57, is a keen golfer and tennis player. In recent years, she has developed right knee pain. For a while, Joanne complains about her "bad knee" but, in general, she ignores it and carries on with what she is doing. She takes lots of magnesium and hot baths, goes through periods of having to rest, and avoids the golf course and tennis court. When she does engage in sport, she often takes painkillers. Eventually, her family gets fed up with her struggle, and urges her to visit her GP. She is referred for an MRI, and learns that her right knee pain is caused by "age-related degeneration".

Joanne is then referred to a physiotherapist, who gives her exercises to strengthen her right hip and thigh muscles to better support her right knee. They also deliver several massages and different high-tech treatments to the right knee area. Joanne feels better for a short while, but then the knee pain comes back. After several cycles of seeing the physio, doing knee strengthening exercises, taking painkillers and receiving some steroid shots to her right knee, Joanne is referred to an orthopaedic surgeon who recommends a knee replacement.

The knee replacement seemingly works for a few years and Joanne carries on playing golf and tennis as before. A few years later, the knee pain returns and now, strangely, the other knee starts to hurt as well. She is told she needs a second knee replacement, so she has another operation. Eventually, the effects of that second knee replacement stop as well and Joanne basically gives up on more surgery, finding it too time consuming, painful and stressful. Sadly, Joanne gives up golf and tennis and never really feels like herself again.

When we change our viewpoint and turn to the Posture Paradigm Shift, we realize that we don't need to suffer in this way. Below is new paradigm in action. I don't personally consider this approach to be new; I think it's just been forgotten. As medicine and technology have improved, I believe our wisdom and common sense have regressed. We rely more and more on other people to fix us using complicated, unnecessary and dramatic interventions, rather than realizing that we are looking for answers in all the wrong places.

FICTIONAL CASE STUDY: FINDING THE ROOT CAUSE

Joanne, aged 57, is a keen golfer and tennis player and has recently developed right knee pain when she plays. Joanne is a logical person and, as with most things, she first applies critical thinking to the cause of this pain. She realizes that her knee pain can't be related to her age because all her joints are the same age. If age were the cause of her pain, then all her joints would hurt in the same way and every person across the world would experience pain in the same way at the same age. She also realizes that her painful knee isn't "bad"; it's a victim of overload and is working too hard. Like a colleague who is taking on double the workload due to a lazy colleague who is not pulling their weight, her painful knee can no longer deal with the extra demand and is starting, quite rightly, to complain. Joanne realizes that something must be happening to her right knee that isn't happening to her left knee.

Joanne visits someone – let's call her Ellie – who looks at the body as a whole and doesn't just consider the right knee as being the only important factor. From looking at Joanne's posture and observing the way Joanne moves, Ellie notices that Joanne is quite rotated forward through her right ribcage, taking her right arm, right shoulder and head along too. Ellie knows that all the parts of the body need to be considered when it comes to weight distribution through the legs and feet, and she realizes that Joanne's right knee hurts because there's significantly more of her upper body twisting over the right side, which means that her right leg is bearing far too much load (fig. 11). The rotated forward upper body position means that Joanne's right knee is taking a battering that the left one is not.

Ellie asks Joanne why she might be rotated like this, and it turns out that Joanne has played tennis and golf for much of her adult life. For a right-handed person like Joanne, both sports require a great deal of right ribcage rotation to occur, and her posture has become a bit stuck like that over the years. By practising several corrective posture exercises that restore the position of her upper body and balance out her right forward ribcage rotation, Joanne frees up her pelvis and hips and brings her weight distribution back to a more centralized position. She walks away from the appointment with absolutely no right knee pain, without ever focusing on the right knee at any point.

Not magic, just logic. The right knee was the messenger; the upper body position was the problem.

The same principle can be applied to almost every single chronic musculoskeletal ache and pain out there, and applying it can create a seemingly miraculous reversal of all sorts of symptoms: arthritis, migraines, neuropathy, disc herniation, hip degeneration, circulation problems, bunions, scoliosis, repetitive strain injuries, lockjaw, tinnitus, vertigo, sciatica, frozen shoulder, blocked sinuses, back pain, neck pain, wrist pain, elbow pain, shoulder pain, foot pain … the list goes on!

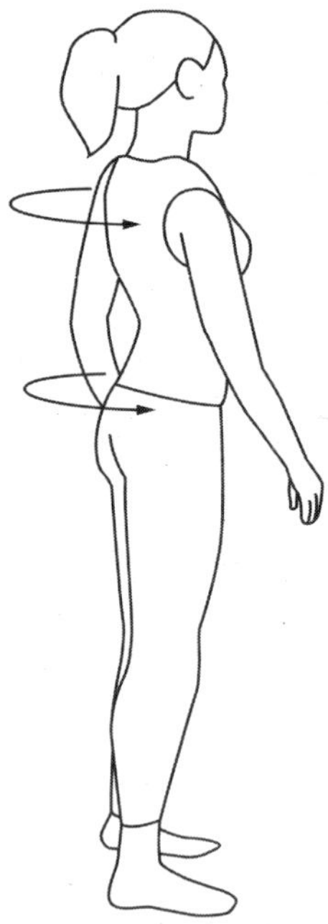

Figure 11: A holistic view of the body shows how right knee pain can be caused by the upper body position overloading the right side.

Later on in the book, in chapter 16, I will give you some practical examples of some of my favourite posture exercises that you can try yourself. Their aim is to reduce rotation in your body (helping with one-sided symptoms like Joanne's), restore your head position back over your shoulders (helping with symptoms like vertigo, migraine, tinnitus, lockjaw, sinus issues and neck pain) and restore pelvic balance (helping with symptoms like sciatica, disc herniation and hip issues).

If you learn to accept and see the body holistically, understand the Posture Paradigm Shift and start to put in the hard work needed to rectify and balance your posture and movement patterns, you will quickly reverse months, years or even decades of pain and tension. It probably is that simple.

For now, we have more theory to explore to motivate you to begin.

TAKEAWAYS

1. Most health care professionals currently focus on symptom suppression and symptom chasing.
2. Pain should be respected, not masked. Pain indicates there is a problem; it is not the problem itself.
3. When we hide from pain and suppress our symptoms, we're not getting the necessary feedback to adapt our behaviour and create helpful change.
4. The area of our body that hurts – the symptom – is most likely not the problem. It's a messenger.
5. The more we focus on the area that hurts – symptom chasing – the more likely we are to aggravate the pain.
6. Symptoms are usually a cry for help: a sign of overwork and exhaustion. By giving an exhausted part of the body even more work to do (with rehab exercises), we are poking the bear and most likely aggravating the symptoms.
7. We need to consider the body as a whole unit, looking at how all the joints and muscles interact. To calm the symptoms, we need to find the parts of us that are not working enough.

CHAPTER SIX

PROBLEM NO. 4: OUR HEALTH IS OUR PROBLEM

We don't become healthy by subcontracting full responsibility to a health care system

The next big problem we face is accountability. Many of us do not take enough responsibility for the choices we make and the role those choices play in ensuring we live our best possible life with the least amount of illness and injury. Admittedly, our modern world works aggressively against our primal needs: without the constant activity and stimulation that comes from building shelters, maintaining fires and finding water and food, making the right decisions for our long-term health becomes more difficult – but it's not impossible. Maintaining a healthy body requires making "boring" choices over a long period of time, such as taking the stairs over the lift, choosing vegetables over ultra-processed foods and prioritizing sleep over late night TV. No one can deny that these choices will slowly stack up to ensure a better quality of life as we age.

I love the quote "if you don't make time for your wellness, you will be forced to make time for your illness,"[16] because good health is generally

If you don't make time for your wellness, you will be forced to make time for your illness.

a result of making the harder choices (short-term pain) for the long-term gains. Bad health is mainly a result of making the easier choices (short-term ease) that result in long-term pain.

While many factors will contribute to the state of our health – such as genetic conditions, traumatic events playing havoc on our nervous system, poverty and not having the luxury of choice, or experiencing a life-changing accident – for most of us, our everyday health is dictated by the everyday choices we make. The food we eat, the water we drink, the sleep we get, the time we spend outdoors, the activities we choose – connecting with people, disconnecting from our electronics, prioritizing true relaxation, reducing stress and so on.

If we make choices that align with the wants and needs of our primal body, we are more likely to end up with better physical and mental health – and vice versa: if we don't align with our primal needs, we will end up with worse health.

This principle brings good news: if it is our choices that most impact our lives, it is fully within the grasp of most of us to create positive change for ourselves. We might not be able to change something 100 per cent, but even a 10 per cent improvement can lead toward a significantly different life. For example, if you were sleeping 10 per cent better (which is one of my favourite side-effects of better posture), that would have a huge knock-on effect on many other aspects of your life: you'd crave less sugar, your hormones would be more stable, your memory would be better, you'd be more clear-headed, you'd be less grumpy and your skin would be brighter.

If we believe the quality of our health is beyond our control, we lose our power and autonomy and we are more likely to feel like a victim of circumstance and poor fortune. We may then succumb to our symptoms and pain, because we don't put in the work to create the changes we need.

Instead, we need to put up a fight!

Aches and pains are not an inevitability. We don't have to sit back and allow them to take over our enjoyment of life, steal our hobbies and sap the energy out of us. To keep aches and pains at bay requires persistence, so if we want to spend our old age doing all the things we love, we have to put up a fight. This is my battle cry to you: you've got to save yourself, because no one else can do it for you. There are many people out there, like me, who can help and support you on your path toward better health, but no one else who can walk that path for you.

Showing yourself self-care and taking responsibility will make you prouder than you can imagine. Believe me, I've been there, and my life has changed beyond recognition since I took responsibility for my actions and my health. I want everyone to experience the confidence that comes with this transformation, because it will change your life for the better in so many ways.

Myth 4: It's my age
We can change our pain if we change our choices

Let's add another posture myth here, to the ones I described in chapter 3. We have all heard someone say, or have maybe said ourselves, something like, "That's just what happens when you get to my age!" or "The doctor says it's age-related degeneration."

I hear this on a frequent basis as a movement teacher and I find it frustrating because I do not believe that ageing causes pain. Not only can I explain this logically, but my experience working with people of all ages supports my theory. In my experience, those of us in our eighties are no less able to reduce our pain than those of us in our twenties. It only comes down to whether we are ready and willing to commit to changing our habits. I bear witness to this every day: all the clients I work with are getting older each day, yet they are still reducing their pain by improving their movement patterns. Here's one such client, going through her perimenopause, which is typically a time when more pain is expected to strike.

"About six years ago, I started to notice my aches and pains becoming increasingly worse. My hips, lower back and upper body felt sore, tired, tight and like they weren't functioning properly. Walking could feel like a chore at times.

I realized that I'm in my perimenopause stage of life and started using HRT and, while this can help, I find Ellie's posture work to be the key to less pain, more mobility and freedom. After finding her, I started to understand how my posture affects my wellbeing.

Since doing the posture work, I feel better. It's a marathon and not a sprint to feel better, and being consistent is key."

Carol

We all age, but ageing does not equate to musculoskeletal pain. In an extremely simplistic nutshell, ageing on a cellular level occurs as an outcome of our cell repair and renewal process becoming more dysfunctional.[17] And, while many of the processes that cause ageing can be slowed down or even reversed,[18] musculoskeletal pain should not factor into the ageing conversation. Musculoskeletal pain is a biomechanical issue.* Biomechanical issues can be caused by accidents, movement habits, breathing patterns, hobbies, holding trauma in the body and stress, but none of these are ageing issues.

I can say this with confidence by looking at the results my clients get, but we can also use data gathered from societies that more similarly replicate the lives of our ancestors.

In modern-day hunter-gatherer societies, the grandparents' vitality is key in providing for their grandchildren, and so

* Except in rare instances when pain could indicate something more sinister, such as a tumour. It is important to consult a medical practitioner to rule out other conditions.

they continue with (what we might consider) remarkable physical feats into their older age. And when I say older age, I do mean older age. Hunter-gatherers who make it past early infancy can, on average, expect to live in good health (that's the important bit) to between 68 and 78 years old.[19] While mothers in the Hadza community in Tanzania are busy tending to their young, the grandparents are working to feed the young, expending, on average, more energy per day in moderate to vigorous activity than the mothers. Generally, Hadza grandmothers forage for five to six hours a day and walk, on average, 8km (5 miles) a day. Hadza grandfathers continue to travel in search of food with the younger men and climb trees to look for fruit and honey.[20]

When measuring the strength of older people in other modern-day hunter-gatherer societies, there is much less physical decline in comparison to their counterparts in Westernized populations.[21] In one study, the grip strength of the average 70-year-old woman of the Aché of Paraguay was similar to the grip strength of the average 50-year-old woman in England.[22] This type of data suggests that the "use it or lose it" principle stands true. Ageing is much less of a problem for those who have always had to be active, and continue to have to be active, to survive.

Using logic, if the ageing process itself did cause musculoskeletal pain, we could assume the following three things without question.

1. All of us would suffer pain in the same places in our body and with the same levels of severity as we age.
2. Each joint in the body is the same age, so all our joints would degenerate identically and at the same time as each other as we age.
3. We wouldn't ever be able to make improvements in how we feel.

Let me debunk this. While it may be common to hear people complain, with increasing amounts of frequency, about their creaky bits as they age, these complaints and their severity differ from person to person.

If ageing caused pain, we would all experience our joints breaking down in the same way, at the same time in our lives and to the same degree. What is really happening is that different muscular dysfunctions and lifestyle factors are playing into the movement patterns that cause pain in different areas of the body for different people.

If ageing caused pain, every part of our body would be in equal amounts of pain as we age. We don't have one knee (for example) that is older than the other, and even if both knees are wearing away and painful, they are still the same age as our shoulders. Logically, we cannot blame the deterioration of one joint or a couple of joints on our age. Something is happening to one particular joint that is not happening to the other joints in your body. Again, it's because of movement patterns and lifestyle.

If ageing caused pain, no one would ever be able to feel better. We would expect a child to recover from the muscle weakness that would occur from resting a broken ankle after falling off a swing, so why not us? We are all experiencing the ageing process, regardless of how old we are. If some of us can improve our muscular function, we can all improve our muscular function. Admittedly, the process will probably take longer the more time your body has had to spiral into dysfunction and the more fixed your neural pathways are. A child will usually make improvements quicker than an adult because they have had less time to lose their muscular function in the first place and the body is closer to remembering what it should be doing. Crucially, children also tend to be more open-minded!

Hope is never lost, and we can always do something about improving our movement patterns. Personally, I'd love for everyone to get into improving their movement patterns as soon as they can – it's so much easier to tackle the biomechanical imbalances before pain or tension sets in –

but there is always the capacity to rebuild muscles[23] and form new habits, even as we get older. You can always teach an "old dog" new postural tricks, if you put the training in.

As I mentioned earlier, I have had clients in their eighties who have significantly reduced their pain through posture exercises. They do the work, they stay committed and they continue to change and challenge their ingrained habits. Please note how I say this in the present tense. Once you start working on your movement patterns, you need to keep doing it. Some of us may stop the posture exercises once our pain has gone, but then are surprised when the pain comes back! To be effective, posture work must become part of your lifestyle, so you continue to keep challenging your muscles and joints.

Regardless of your age, as you start working on your posture and waking up your muscles, you'll release compression from your hip joints, unwind twisting in your knee joints, lift the arches of your flat feet, reposition your shoulders behind you and learn to breathe through your diaphragm. You'll notice your pain and tension reducing. At this point, you'll no longer be able to blame your age for causing your pain, because you are still, of course, ageing, but your pain and tension are lessening.

But if ageing doesn't cause pain, why do so many people suffer pain as they get older?

TAKEAWAYS

1. You must take responsibility for your own health and the choices you make.
2. Subcontracting your health out to someone else will never grow your confidence and intuition.
3. You are the only person who can truly create change for yourself.

4. Age does not cause pain. We can deduce this logically and by using data from modern-day hunter-gatherer societies.
5. You can always change how well your muscles work, and so you can always change how you feel – regardless of your age.
6. Changing habits is the biggest contributing factor to reducing musculoskeletal pain.

CHAPTER SEVEN
THE ACTUAL CAUSES OF MUSCULOSKELETAL PAIN

It's time to see things differently

There is a fundamental difference between causation and correlation, and we can easily get them mixed up when it comes to pain and ageing.

To help you understand this principle, I want to use an unrelated example. If studied, I am sure we could find a correlation between people taking off their jumpers and the sales of ice creams in the summer. Both things happen alongside an increase in heat and sunshine (the causation). But it would be madness to think that the act of taking off a jumper causes a magical surge in the sale of ice creams, right? That would clearly not be considering all the relevant factors and would be falsely attributing a causation – rather than seeing both actions as correlated to another factor (the heat of the sun). The thought that age causes pain is as illogical as thinking taking your jumper off increases ice cream sales.

We are not looking carefully enough at the bigger picture when it comes to age and pain, and so are missing a key variable. Age is the purchase of ice creams and pain is taking off a jumper. The variety and frequency of our movement patterns and how we have maintained these over our lives make up the crucial variable (the sun). I'm no mathematician, but I hope I can use some equations to demonstrate this more clearly.

Incorrect equation (missing the key variable)

$$\uparrow A = \uparrow P$$

Increasing age = increasing pain

Potentially correct equations (including the key variable)

1. $$\uparrow A + \downarrow QM = \uparrow P$$

Increasing age + decreasing quality, variety and frequency of movement patterns = increasing pain

2. $$\uparrow A + \uparrow QM = XP$$

Increasing age + maintaining or increasing quality, variety and frequency of movement patterns = staying pain-free

Therefore ...

$$\uparrow A = \uparrow P \quad \text{for you} \quad \uparrow QM = \downarrow P$$

If you are experiencing increasing pain as you age, you must increase your quality of movement in order to decrease this pain.

I like to think of our life, body and movement patterns as a length of string (fig. 16). For every sedentary year that passes, for each muscle that seizes up and becomes dysfunctional, for every accident we have and for every stressful event that happens, we add a knot to our string. Posture work slowly unravels these knots. Children tend to have fewer knots in their string than adults. This isn't because adults' bodies are older physically, but because they have had more time to potentially pick up trauma and dysfunctional movement habits. Some people stay active, mobile, healthy and relaxed their whole lives and accumulate few knots along the way. You only need to look at images of 100-year-old yoga gurus still twisting themselves into challenging poses for proof. These people are in the minority, but they show how a mobile body can be maintained into old age with the right stimulus.

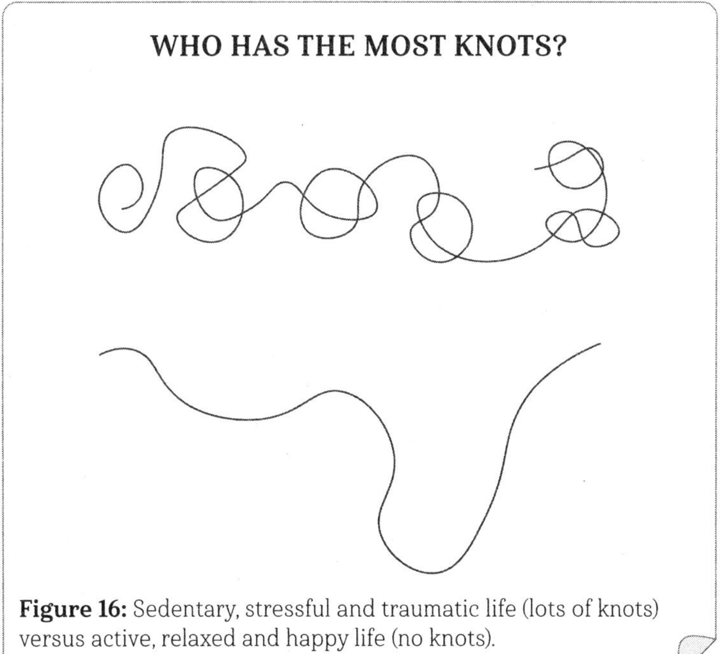

Figure 16: Sedentary, stressful and traumatic life (lots of knots) versus active, relaxed and happy life (no knots).

> Hypothetically, either length of string could belong to a 15-year-old or a 50-year-old. It is more likely that the 50-year-old will have more knots, but it's not a definite. You may be an active relaxed 50-year-old who has not experienced much trauma, has always maintained a physically active (including varied movement) life and has managed to stay knot-free. Or you may be a 15-year-old who has had a stressful upbringing, with a lot of sedentary video gaming and several dramatic acute accidents (such as a serious fall), and has developed a lot of knots, very young. The age isn't the determining factor; it's what happens during your life that matters.

Some examples of how we might reduce pain, regardless of age, include:

- Changing how sedentary we are and moving more frequently
- Learning to regulate our nervous system
- Learning how to breathe functionally
- Restoring function to each muscle in our body
- Restoring mobility to each joint in our body

As you work on your posture, you'll realize there is no causation between age and pain, only correlation.

In my opinion, the actual causation of pain is the life-long degradation of three movement-related factors.

1. How much we move
2. How well we move
3. How varied our movement is

Let's look at these three causes of musculoskeletal pain in more detail.

Cause 1: It's going wrong from day one
Our environment and modern technologies stop us from moving enough

The human body is a powerful and resilient machine that is designed to move frequently or most of the day. Indeed, it is through frequent movement and physical challenge that we stay powerful and resilient, both in body and mind. Sadly, for many of us, our idea of what constitutes a "normal" daily movement level differs greatly from how much movement we need to thrive.

On a typical working day, I guess that many of us are awake for about 16 hours a day and that around 9 to 13 of those hours are spent sitting down:[24] commuting, working at a desk, commuting, relaxing on the sofa. Ouch, not good!

Let's take stock of how long we follow this pattern of behaviour. For a typical desk worker, this will probably be your routine for decades, while you serve your time in the working world. On top of that, let's consider how our modern childhood movement patterns don't differ much from this post-industrial model of living. This means that our muscles and bones are being disrupted from infancy.

The wonderful anthropologist and movement teacher Esther Gokhale makes a great point that modern industrial societies create splintered family units, which often means geographical separation between grandchildren and grandparents. The ancient wisdom and "kinaesthetic traditions" (the ability to know where the parts of your body are and how they are moving) of how to correctly hold, feed and exercise a baby to improve their muscular development used to be passed down through close-knit generations, but this tradition has slowly withered away.[25]

Our muscular degradation begins from the moment we are born, thanks to various forms of modern technology. Baby bottles impact the formation of our jaw and face muscles,[26] and we are put in car seats, baby bouncers, playpens, nappies, restrictive shoes, highchairs, pushchairs and baby walkers. All these modern devices, and more, are stripping away our movement, deforming our posture[27] and warping the development and correct sequencing of our movement patterns.

Now, I need to caveat, I am not a parent, and I am not here to judge anyone's parenting. But I am here to tell you a few (possibly difficult) home truths about some supposedly normal things in our modern environment that are anything but normal for our bodies. I firmly believe that awareness breeds power and change, and so we need to hear and understand this type of thing.

We need to let a baby's muscles develop in the right order. Until very recently, in the grand course of human history – and without pushchairs (invented in 1733 and only popularized when they become more affordable in the late 1890s)[28] and other modern devices mentioned above – most babies spent most of their time being held in someone's arms[29] or strapped to their mother's body.[30] Being strapped to another human is not only good for a baby's security and comfort, but it's also great for opening the baby's hips and developing a strong spine, because it requires constant muscular readjustment and stabilization from the baby. Much like how sitting on a wobbly Pilates ball is good for our muscles, so is being strapped to another moving being while you can't move on your own.[31]

Laying a baby on a flat surface (rather than propping them in a seat), and leaving them to their own movement devices, allows the muscles of the body to develop in the "right order", typically from the inside out. Our deepest postural muscles are with us at birth, and the most surface level (superficial) muscles develop over several years, waymarked by movement milestones. In a typical movement journey, first comes the supine (lying flat) flailing about of the limbs, then the roll to the tummy (prone), then the sitting position, then the push to the hands and knees (quadruped), then the crawl, then the first tentative steps, and then the stand.[32] Typically, the steady standing position occurs after some walking, because moving using momentum is easier than standing still. Each of these milestones denotes a new level of muscular development and, if a baby is handled correctly and not placed in a never-ending sequence of chairs, things will happen at nature's pace and order. If we interfere too much with the movement development process, a baby will bypass certain milestones, and those missing pieces can impact their life-long biomechanics and proprioception (also known as kinaesthesia).[33]

Modern baby equipment interferes with a baby's musculoskeletal development. I believe that putting a baby in a seat that props them up and holds them still for a long period of time, before they can do it themselves using muscular strength, disrupts nature's order. By strapping a baby in a seat, or propping a young child in a chair to eat or watch TV, we strip their body of muscular demand. And as you know by now, it is through frequent demand that our muscles become strong.

We also use other modern items that interrupt or scramble the development of a baby's muscles and bones. For example, by putting a baby in a pair of firm shoes (such as Doc Martens, Crocs or any shoe with a thick stiff sole), it allows them to stand earlier, perhaps before their body is ready. For a baby to stand up barefoot, they need a lot of coordination, balance and strength through their core, pelvis, legs and feet. But it's much easier to stand up in a stiff pair of shoes, and a baby needs a lot less coordination, balance and strength to achieve this stance. This isn't a good thing, because it is interrupting the natural order of muscular and bone development and it is encouraging our children to do too much, too soon. We need our deep, intrinsic, core muscular development to happen in the right order as a child to retain strong resilient muscles and joints into adulthood.

Baby bouncers and baby walkers allow a baby to artificially "move" beyond their capabilities (while also trapping them in a supported seated position). These products take the work that should be happening in the muscles of the baby's feet and legs and subcontract that work into the bouncer or walker. So much of our crucial development happens before the age of 18, and it's extremely important that we are physically challenged in our very early years. If we are, we will have greater musculoskeletal robustness in later life.[34]

Sitting still for long periods at school impacts our physical and social development. Not only do our modern babyhoods disrupt our body's development and mess with our idea of "normal", but so does our schooling system. As early as the late 19th century, when it became increasingly common for children to receive an education, concerns were already mounting about what the post-industrial schooling system was doing to the developing bodies and minds of children: "With his introduction to school life, the child's physical troubles begin. He is made to sit still from 3 to 6 hours, with but momentary rests at long intervals, [and] the play instinct, expressed by recurrent attacks of the 'fidgets' has to be sternly suppressed by the teacher for the sake of discipline."[35]

I believe that our schooling system keeps children sitting still for far too long during some of their most crucial and impactful periods of both physical and mental development. While children may get play breaks and physical education lessons, it is not enough movement to optimize and support their development. Unrestricted physical play with peers not only keeps us physically strong, but it also helps us develop social skills, boundaries, a sense of what is right and wrong, resilience, problem solving, independence, quick thinking, imagination[36] – the list goes on. How many of these critical life skills can you develop from sitting still all day looking at a whiteboard or screen?

On a more profound level, our lack of movement messes with our self-expression. Many of us are taught from a young age that "good children" sit still and don't fidget. If we get told off for running around and playing, we quickly learn that sitting still and being quiet is the route to an easier life. This means we are being emotionally blackmailed in some of our earliest years to go entirely against our slightly wild, primal, human nature, to conform to what makes sense in our capitalist world.

With his introduction to school life, the child's physical troubles begin.

For some of you, I hope I have helped illustrate how each stage of your life has probably worked against the development of your muscles and your natural innate human resilience. Many of the things I have described in this chapter were entirely out of your control, and not the fault of your parents either. Yet again, the issue is our societal disconnection from the environment in which we originally evolved. Awareness breeds power, and I hope the points I have made help shape some small everyday decisions for future parenting. If you want my advice, keep your baby out of sitting devices and shoes as much and for as long as possible. As a general rule of thumb, if your baby can't do a movement by themselves, they shouldn't be propped or held in that position for any length of time. Also, lead by example and try and move as much as you can yourself.

For others of you, I suspect nothing I have said here is new. Many of us are fully aware of the restrictions our modern environment places on our health, our childhood development and our ongoing muscular strength, and many of us are already trying to do something to combat the epidemic of sedentarism. Exercise. Unfortunately, many of our typical exercise choices are also the causes of much of our pain.

Cause 2: We move, but we don't move well
We are inadvertently causing our pain

We tend to be a society of "weekend warriors". We spend most of our time at a desk, in a car or on a sofa (and have done for decades), but will then do as much exercise as we can in the time we have available – often the weekend. Gyms, running clubs and yoga studios are full of enthusiastic (yet frequently injured) clients trying their hardest to get their heart pumping, body sweating and muscles aching, wanting to stay strong. So, what is going wrong?

I think the issue was nicely articulated by orthopaedist Walter Truslow in 1943: "We are forever engaging in activities which tend toward asymmetry and derangement of our architecture."[37] And, because the architecture of our body is compromised, high-intensity exercise causes imbalanced load through the joints, leading to wear and tear and tension.

The problem is that many of us tend to focus solely on the intensity of our exercise, not the variety and quality of our movement. Let me explain what I mean by this. We know that our body needs to sweat, our heart needs to pump and our muscles need to be challenged to stay strong. However, most of us are so time-poor and exhausted that there is normally only a small window in the day (or week) to do these things. We focus on trying to do as much (often quite high-intensity) exercise as possible in a short space of time, without considering what our body is designed to do movement-wise, and how we are performing the exercise we have chosen.

The construct of exercise is a modern phenomenon. Historical sources suggest that ancient warriors exercised with intention, to keep themselves battle-ready through physical activity like wrestling, sprinting and javelin throwing.[38] They did not exercise for fun or for the health benefits, rather to be good at their job. Beyond this, everyday folk probably didn't exercise formally or deliberately. Yes, there were public dances, races, sports and competitions (going back thousands of years), but these events were not aimed at losing weight or maintaining health, nor were they participated in by most regular people. Such events were to demonstrate athletic prowess and achieve pride over neighbouring towns and villages, for entertainment in a pre-TV world or to reach some form of spiritual state. These types of ancient rituals, sports and tournaments are a far cry from us pounding out an hour on the treadmill to offset our desk time or to lose weight.

Not that long ago, people didn't need to exercise for their health because they moved enough through necessity. We only really started sitting still for work en masse during the boom of the Industrial Revolution, so it was only then that the truly sedentary working day set in and the concept of exercise as we know it emerged.

Prior to this time, life would have been hard work and active in a near-constant, low-level type of way. Our ancestors 500 years ago wouldn't have been doing kipping on pull-up bars or jumping up and down doing lunges, but they would have been strong from chopping wood, tying ropes, carrying buckets, walking everywhere and squatting in the fields to pick crops. We are designed to stay gently active for most of the day, with some occasional spells of high-intensity action such as responding to an attack or sprinting to hunt down an animal. This gentle constant action throughout life would have kept the body primed for the short bursts of high-intensity action needed. Our normal lives were once the training ground for our muscles.

Even the masses of people who left farming for the allure of the city factories 200 or so years ago would have led significantly more active lives than we do today. Despite many of the roles in factories being extremely stationary (in comparison to the work performed on farms or hunting and gathering), people probably travelled to work on foot and had to do a lot more physical labour to maintain the household – in the absence of supermarkets, washing machines and vacuum cleaners.

It is only as our lives have become even more stationary that the need for and construct of exercise has really developed. However, an hour a day (at best for most of us) cannot mitigate the other 15 waking hours of being still. In studies, those of us who exercise frequently but who also spend a lot of time sitting down are 60 per cent more susceptible to inflammatory related diseases than those of us who are less fit, but sit less.[39] Even if we engage in more than seven hours per week of moderate to vigorous exercise, but continue to sit a lot, we are still 50 per cent more likely to die from cardiovascular disease.[40] The whole premise of modern-day exercise is short sighted, because it is trying to make our human physiology fit into the wrong-shaped box. Square peg, round hole. Our bodies stay healthy and robust through frequent gentle movement all day, not an aggressive hour or so every now and then. Short bursts of intense movement practice, within the context of extreme sedentarism, are out of alignment with our nature and work against achieving optimal health.

Aside from the musculoskeletal mismatch between our biological design and our modern exercise culture, I think there is a real point to be made about how many of us have exercise regimes that work against our fatigued mental state and dysregulated nervous system. We live in a world of constant bustle and stress, and the high-intensity workouts we cram in can raise cortisol levels, increase dysfunctional breathing patterns and make the body more prone to inflammation, injury and exhaustion. The more stress we suffer, the worse we sleep, the more sugar and caffeine we crave, and the more bloated and inflamed our body is. If we are stressed out and depleted, shouldn't movement mainly serve to calm and ground us rather than wind us up even more?

How we exercise is important. Many of us do not stop to think about the sedentary body and stiff imbalanced posture we are bringing to our workouts. A hunter-gatherer, who spends their whole life staying active for most of the day, would probably be able to perform high-intensity workouts quite easily and without harm. Their whole lifestyle is a training ground for higher intensity activity. But our modern lifestyle is, instead, a training ground for muscular weakness, imbalanced joints, wear and tear in the bones and a losing battle against gravity. We need to think about *how* we exercise.

As we have already established, if we sit still for most of the day, our muscles become weak and our body becomes stiff. A yoga or gym class may make us more flexible and stronger than some of our colleagues in the office, but it won't make us flexible or strong compared to what would have been normal human muscular function a few thousand years ago. Our muscles fall asleep as we sit in a chair, our crossed legs pull our hips, spine and pelvis out of alignment; our heavy head and shoulders dangle in front of our laptop pulling down our spine; our bones, tendons and ligaments lose the protection and support that strong muscles provide; and everything starts to collapse in on itself and wear away. We create extremely unstable foundations that are unsuitable for high-intensity activity.

We shouldn't try to run before we can walk. Most of us are severely underprepared physically for the types of exercise we are trying to do. We are expecting our bodies to respond positively to sitting still most of the time and then being physically beaten up in a strength class or during a long run a couple of times a week. Because of our sedentary lifestyle, we need to consciously prepare our body for this level of demand. We need to restore our basic levels of muscular function, balance our joints and free up compression between our bones before asking our body to do things it is vastly ill equipped to handle. We are trying to run long distances with hips that are bound up from decades of sitting, we are trying to swing golf clubs with ribcages and shoulders that are too stiff to rotate, and we are trying to contort ourselves into challenging poses and arm balances in a yoga class with a body that is all out of whack. And then we wonder why our physical pursuits often cause us tension, pain and injury.

Balanced and functional high-intensity exercise is incredibly good for the joints. Imbalanced and dysfunctional exercise is incredibly bad for the joints. Preparation, effort and practice are key to achieving balanced and functional movement patterns that do not damage our joints or create tension in our muscles. To stay pain-free while moving, we must restore the basic foundations of movement and mobility first, before we attack the gym, running club or yoga studio. We may have to take some time away from our favourite activities, especially if they are ones that cause frequent injury and tension, but the postural groundwork we put in instead will reap so many long-term rewards.

To those of you who baulk at the idea of temporarily giving up a beloved sport or hobby while you repair your movement patterns, ask yourself how much more you will enjoy your hobby when you are no longer having to deal with recurring injuries and tension. How amazing will it feel to continue your activity for many years longer than your contemporaries who didn't invest in repairing their movement patterns? And how exciting will it be to move so efficiently that you are faster, stronger or more flexible than you have ever been?

For many of us, we are missing the middleman of exercise, and it's damaging us. We are an all or nothing culture: either sat still at a desk/in a car/on a sofa or trying to run a marathon. Where's the in between? How have we arrived at a point where those of us who can't stand upright against a wall for a few minutes (remember our posture test earlier?) are furiously training to conquer an Ironman triathlon?

MOVEMENT PROFILE

Now, don't get me wrong. I am not dismissing the importance of raising our heartbeat, getting a sweat on, making our muscles scream with effort and loading our joints with more intensity against the forces of gravity.[41] High-intensity exercise is certainly important, but it should not comprise most of our movement profile, especially if we spend most of the day being still. The largest portion of our movement profile, if we are looking to best replicate the movement of hunter-gatherers, should involve gently engaging in varied tasks and movements that keep our bodies supple and strong. Things like household chores, gardening, carrying bags, walking and posture exercises are far more likely to help us move in the way we should than daily long runs or going to the gym five times a week.

Cause 3: Not enough movement variety
Repetitive movement patterns create wear and tear

All the muscles in the body need to be taken through their full ranges of movement on a regular basis to stay functional and to hold our joints in an efficient comfortable position. As mentioned previously, the more functional all our muscles are, the less musculoskeletal pain we will experience. If we were living the life for which our body was designed, we would be exercising every single part of us without even realizing. For example, the dexterity and strength of our hands would stay consistently challenged with actions like foraging and crafting tools. Our spine and hips would not have seized up because we would not be sitting down in passive hip and spinal flexion. Our hips would be kept mobile through walking, squatting and some occasional bouts of running. Our feet wouldn't be strangled and deformed by pointed or heeled shoes, and our toes, mid-feet, ankles and calves would be powerful and supportive for the rest of our body. Our shoulders would be kept mobile by chopping wood, hunting with a bow and arrow and washing our clothes by hand. And our eyes and facial muscles would be kept busy through the constant stimulation of the senses – not tired, drooping, sagging, wrinkling and lifeless in front of a screen. Life would, without much thought, be keeping every single joint and muscle in our body regularly challenged in a variety of ways.

Modern life does not do this. It has proactively stripped varied challenge and function away from our joints and muscles. And to compound these issues of weakness, stiffness and dysfunction, many types of exercise often focus on working certain muscles in certain monotonous ranges of motion, which can lead to further stiffness and pain.

Take cycling for example. The posture of a cyclist is one of repetitive pelvic flexion, spinal flexion, rounded shoulders and forward head (fig. 17). While the heart will beat fast and the legs will pump (moving between knee and hip flexion and knee and hip extension as we pedal), few individual parts of the body are moving and being challenged. The macro-parts of the cyclist are being transported to a different location, but the micro-parts of the body itself aren't moving with much variety. The hips are only really moving through flexion and extension, with little need for rotation, adduction and abduction. The pelvis is generally locked in a tucked, flexed, posterior pelvic tilt, which switches off many of the muscles around the hips and spine. While on a bike leaning forward, the flexed C-shape spine does not get the chance to extend, rotate or laterally flex, and the shoulders are stuck in a hunched rounded position without being asked to extend, rotate, abduct or retract. And normally the head of a cyclist is dangling in front of the shoulders and the hands are locked stiffly in a claw shape on the handlebars. Cycling may be good cardio exercise, but it does not encourage varied movement patterns and cannot really be said to be too productive for your posture

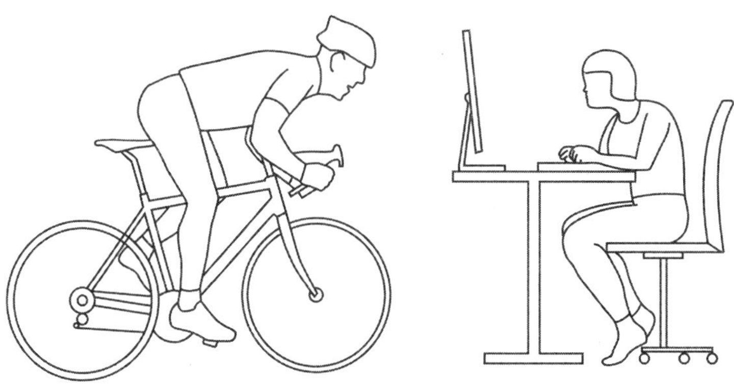

Figure 17: Flexion while cycling versus flexion while sitting. How different are these postures really?

And, not to demonize cycling too much (there are plenty of other types of exercise that are also repetitive and monotonous for our joints), but cycling almost perfectly mimics the sedentary position we are already locked in for many hours of the day (fig. 17). The person who cycles regularly but does few other forms of movement, is most likely strengthening the stiff seated position their posture is already locked in. Being strong in a locked-up and stiff position is not a recipe for staying pain-free. Being mobile through all sorts of varied joint positions is.

TAKEAWAYS

1. We are not moving enough. From the moment we are born, our movement patterns are dramatically impacted and altered by modern technology.
2. Modern technology and modern lifestyles affect the quantity, variety and quality of our movement and can warp our sense of normal human movement.
3. We invented the construct of exercise to mitigate how little our modern lives require us to move.
4. Many of us are trying to do too much in a short space of time. The human body has evolved for lots of gentle, more constant movement throughout the day with occasional bouts of high intensity.
5. Many of us are trying to exercise too vigorously in a body that has adapted to sedentarism, without restoring muscular function and joint balance first. We are, therefore, causing our own pain and injury.
6. Many forms of exercise are extremely repetitive and do not offer each muscle and each joint the requisite ranges of motion needed to maintain musculoskeletal health.

CHAPTER EIGHT
THE RIGHT TYPE OF MOVEMENT

What does the body require to stay pain-free?

All the causes of musculoskeletal pain I have mentioned so far are interlinked. However, because of the way many of us approach exercise, we are probably ignoring the most important part of our movement patterns. If our goal is to be mobile and stay pain-free, we should be asking ourselves the following question:

"Have I moved every single joint and muscle in my body through its full range of movement recently?"

And when I say every single joint and muscle, I mean *every* single joint and muscle. Because the body is connected throughout its entire structure via a web of muscles, bones, ligaments, tendons and fascia, every single part of it is extremely important. Think of your body as a vast orchestra in which each musician plays their part in performing a perfect symphony. The violinist may do more than the bassoonist, but you'd miss the presence of the bassoon if the orchestra didn't have one.

Maintaining the movement of your fingers and toes is no less important than maintaining the strength of your glutes and biceps. Preserving the strength and mobility of your ankles and wrists is no less important than doing the same for your spine and hips. Sustaining the movement of your eyes, the strength of your jaw muscles and the power of your diaphragm to breathe functionally is no less important than getting defined abs or pecs. Many of us concentrate too hard on the surface-level muscles we think will improve our aesthetic, at the expense of all the deep important muscles we cannot see. Our goal is often to improve how we look rather than how we feel, but it is whole body muscular function that keeps us pain-free. Ironically, the more efficiently our body moves – which happens because of improved muscular function and more balanced joints – the more our muscles are stimulated during even gentle movement, and so can naturally tone themselves and become more muscular with far less effort.

I know looking good can be a powerful motivator, and there is nothing wrong with that if it helps you make time to work on your posture. When we are only moving, perhaps inadvertently, some parts of us (rather than all parts), we will notice stubborn fleshy bits that are hard to tone or areas that seem out of proportion with other bits. For example, you'll see a big heavy-lifting gym-goer with tiny calves or a muscular yogi with defined abs but a flat bum. The calves aren't naturally tiny, nor does the yogi naturally have a flat bum. Those are the parts of the body that are not being moved enough, relative to other areas. They are understimulated and are not receiving enough demand to stay toned and proportionate in size. Personally, I struggle with wobbly rear upper arms and fleshy cellulite-ridden hamstrings. This isn't my natural lot; it's that my triceps and my hamstrings are less functional than other parts of me. They are not being used enough as I move and are, therefore, less toned. As a posture therapist, it's quite easy to spot someone's dysfunctional and compensating areas of the body purely on visuals alone. Muscular tone and size (as well as joint positioning) tell me a lot about what is overworking (compensating) and what is underworking (dysfunctional).

As I briefly mentioned earlier, your posture holds your face together, too. If the face muscles are not being stimulated enough, because you spend too much time indoors and looking at a screen, your eyes will be weaker and your face will be more droopy and more asymmetrical than it should be. If your head is dangling in front of your shoulders (eventually getting "stuck" there), the skin on the neck will become more wrinkly and saggy than it should be. Your posture doesn't just impact your torso and limbs, it impacts the position of your facial features, too. Almost everything is controlled by muscles.

We need a good range of movement

Hopefully, I have explained why we need to exercise all the joints and muscles in the body. Now let's look at range of movement.

As demonstrated in our cycling example in chapter 7, it is not enough to merely move a body part. We must also consider how we move that body part and what it has the capability to do: its range of movement. For example, if we wear shoes with arch support and marginal heels (such as a normal trainer or walking boot), our foot is stuck in a perpetual state of plantarflexion (pointing downward). Due to the raised heel in the shoe, the foot is not able to achieve proper dorsiflexion (pulling backward of the foot) during the gait cycle, and the arch support is taking away the foot's ability to pronate and supinate in the mid-foot properly. So, even though the foot is moving, it is not moving through its full range of movement (more on feet and footwear later in this chapter; pages 106–129).

At this point, you may be thinking, which exercise or sport will give me everything I need movement wise? I'd argue that no one type of exercise or sport will give you absolutely everything you require, but well-performed yoga comes close – from a range of movement standpoint.* The reason

* By "well-performed", I mean yoga performed with enough muscular function and body awareness. Many of us try to do yoga when we do not have enough muscular function to really benefit from the poses, and so there's a lot of imbalance and compensation occurring. In this case, yoga is likely to lead toward more pain and injury.

yoga is difficult for many of us (at first, at least) is because it requires more joint mobility, control and function than most other forms of exercise. It works on and builds a type of strength that regular gym classes don't tend to focus on. But the extra mobility gained from yoga is, in my opinion, the type of physical strength that will keep you pain-free for longest. The difficult poses and balances that seasoned yogis can perform are achievable because they have retained or regained their muscular function and joint mobility, not because they are simply naturally bendy. However, yoga isn't perfect. If we want a good range of movement, yoga is missing a few important elements: high intensity, heavy gravitational load and explosive power – plus, arguably, there's not much of a "pulling" motion in yoga postures. In my opinion, if we are looking to stay pain-free for as long as possible, we are better off becoming movement generalists (like our ancestors) and not specializing too hard in one thing.

Improving your posture will help set the foundations for other exercise or sport. By doing your corrective posture exercises, strengthening your dysfunctional muscles, improving the range of motion at every joint in your body, learning how to breathe functionally and balancing your joints, you set up your body for success. If you include posture exercises in your daily schedule, you won't need to ask yourself "Have I moved every single joint in my body through its full range of movement recently?" And you'll be able to get on with your favourite activities without much thought, with better results and far less injury. The cyclist with the desk job isn't going to have as many issues with stiffness and pain if they simultaneously invest time in restoring their overall mobility by doing posture exercises regularly. They'll also cycle faster and longer than ever before. Efficient muscular and joint function is an incredibly powerful thing.

Myth 5: Gravity is the enemy
Do our joints wear away because of gravity?

Now seems a good time to unpick another posture myth. Sometimes, I hear things like "Running is bad for your joints" or "Our spines aren't designed to keep us upright properly so lower back pain is inevitable". If you think about it, these ideas are based on the notion that the body is not designed to cope with the forces of gravity, and that our joints and bodies instead need protection from gravity.

I suggest this is the wrong way of looking at things. I believe that maintaining your body's ability to tussle regularly against the forces of gravity is hugely important in staying pain-free, robust and strong in your muscles and your bones – especially as you age.

Most of us can probably accept that gravity has been present for the whole of human evolution. Therefore, we can, I think, safely assume that humans learned to stand on two legs in an environment that was always fighting against gravity. This would suggest that we are designed to constantly interact with gravity. So, when our bodies are taken out of an environment with gravitational load, we struggle. We know that when astronauts go into space, their muscle mass diminishes by 20 per cent in two weeks.[42] We also know that running (under the full weight of Earth's gravitational pull) helps to promote healthy joint cartilage and protects against osteoarthritis[43] and that runners, therefore, tend to have better bone density than cyclists and swimmers.[44]

Additionally, research has revealed that the more we load our bones in the first 20 years of life, the thicker they are[45] and the less prone to osteoarthritis we are as we age.[46] And, as our society has become more sedentary, conditions like osteoarthritis and osteoporosis have become more common.[47] All of these things, and many more, heavily suggest that our muscles and joints are kept strong *because* of their constant tussle with gravity, not despite it.

Human bone density has changed significantly since our move away from the gravitational rigours of a hunter-gatherer lifestyle and into a relatively more sedentary lifestyle, afforded to our ancestors by agricultural developments. Even 7,000 years ago (well into the Agricultural Revolution), it's likely that the average woman had bones that were 30 per cent stronger than those of the average woman today, meaning a typical farming woman had better bone density than most current-day athletes.[48] That's quite the degradation!

What's going wrong? We aren't interacting with gravity enough anymore because of our sedentary lifestyles, cushioned shoes, soft beds and comfy chairs (which make our muscles switch off). These modern factors impact our body, which then begins to struggle with the forces of gravity. In turn, we may withdraw from activities that challenge our joints under the forces of gravity, because we are too sedentary, and so gravitationally loaded exercises often cause us pain.

Think of things like jumping, skipping, dancing, running and even walking. These gravitationally loaded forms of exercise require our body to be able to efficiently combat the forces of gravity. When we perform these higher intensity types of activities, there is a vertical force of gravity fighting against the firmness of the floor. Our body is sandwiched in the middle, and our joints and muscles are absorbing the shock between the two forces. The harder our legs push down into the floor, the harder the ground pushes back. This is Newton's third law of motion in action,[49] and this is gravitational load being put through the joints of our body.

Think of things like cycling, swimming, yoga and Pilates as less-loaded forms of exercise that do not require our body to work against gravity so much. In these examples, your joints are not having to work as shock absorbers to the same degree, because there's much less of a fight between gravity, the floor and your body. However, within these types of exercise, there is nuance, because, for example, off-road mountain biking puts a lot more gravitational force through your body than road biking on a flat surface.[50] Both forms of cycling are involving more or less the same body movement, but that movement is happening within a different environment and, therefore, creating different interactions with gravity.

A regular fight between your body, the ground and the force of gravity toughens your bones and joints. We already understand the concept that our muscles become denser and stronger through repeated regular demand and load on them. For example, at the gym, challenging the muscles by lifting increasingly heavier weights over time will tear the fibres of the muscles. The muscles then repair these torn fibres and, in doing so, they lay down more muscle fibres and become bigger in size and stronger in capability.

Our bones and joints are the same, and they need regular demanding gravitational load to become denser and stronger. The more our bones are asked to act as shock absorbers during higher intensity exercise, the denser and more resilient they become. However, for many of us, higher intensity exercise is problematic and causes joint pain. If our bodies are designed to fight against gravity like I say, why are we experiencing pain?

Perhaps you already know what I am about to say. The answer is: many of us struggle to remain pain-free because we have dysfunctional imbalanced movement patterns. Our joints' response to gravity would be a different story if we reacquired our mobile posture, balanced our joints and became more functional in our movement patterns.

Balanced, aligned, functional bodies respond well to higher intensity exercise and gravity. Balanced and aligned joints are able to act as the pain-free shock absorbers they are designed to be, because they are being held in biomechanically efficient positions. When our bodies move functionally, we can leap off a high wall and land heavily in a squat, we can run for a long distance, and we can jump up and down on the dancefloor – and feel great while doing so.

Imbalanced, misaligned, dysfunctional bodies struggle with higher intensity exercise and gravity. Imbalanced and misaligned joints cannot act as pain-free shock absorbers, because they are not being held in biomechanically efficient positions. For each joint that is not in balance and able to hold the human structure in the most efficient and balanced way (as per its evolutionary blueprint), the overloading joints are going to begin to wear away.

In figure 18, one of the bodies loves its fight with gravity and the other struggles with joint pain and muscular tension. The pain may be enough for the person to begin to withdraw from activities that load the bones. Not hard to guess which is which.

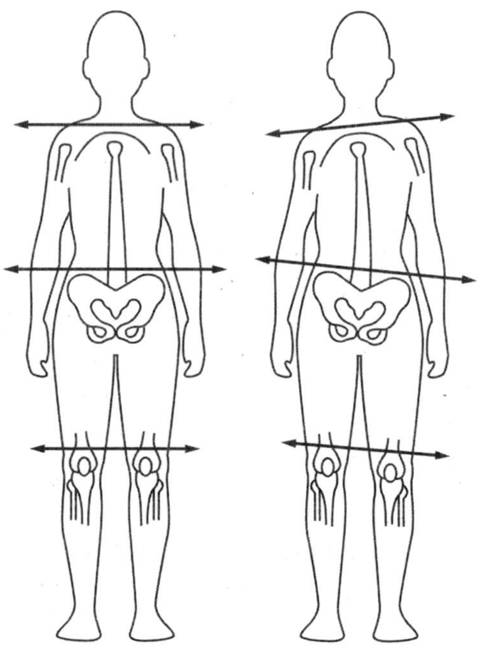

Figure 18: Balance versus imbalance. In an aligned body gravity bears equal load through the joints, but in a misaligned body gravity bears too much load through some joints, but not others.

Tale as old as time. We all know the runner who struggles with increasing levels of knee pain. Eventually, they may replace their running with Nordic walking, but then Nordic walking starts to hurt their knees, too. They then try cycling, but cycling begins to hurt their back and so they switch to swimming. By the time they are swimming as their only form of exercise, their body is barely having to perform its natural fight against gravity at all, and this only weakens the density of their bones. As the bones lose density, the body becomes more brittle and more susceptible to injury. The more susceptible to injury we become, the longer we must spend resting and staying still. This leads to more muscular weakness and then more pain. Hopefully, you can see the chain of events. If we avoid interacting with gravity, it doesn't only impact bone density but also our whole body movement ability.

If we want to prevent the onset of conditions like osteoporosis, avoiding gravitational loading because it causes us pain is a serious problem. Higher intensity exercise is important throughout our entire lifetime – not just something we should be doing as children and young adults. We must consider our ability to continue to perform higher intensity exercise pain-free as a demonstration of how balanced our joints are. If we are not able to fight against gravity pain-free, we must work hard to restore and improve our posture and movement patterns until we are sufficiently balanced and functional to do higher intensity exercise again. Ideally, we don't ever want to lose this ability, because, by the time you lose it, it will require a lot more time and work to gain it back. Retain your ability to perform higher intensity exercise throughout your life and things will be a lot easier for you.

Myth 6: Our bodies need support
Is the human body not fit for purpose?

In my opinion, this myth is hugely connected to the misconception that the human body doesn't work synergistically with gravity. I know that many of us think that our body needs protecting. For example, recently I went to a gong bath (they're great – look it up!) and heard a comment from the percussionist that made my toes curl, "Our bodies aren't designed to lie on a hard floor for long periods of time." In my view, this person had lost some perspective, because humans have slept on the floor, without bedding as we know it, for most of human history.[51] However, the percussionist is not alone in their view: many of us seem to think that our bodies are somehow not fit for purpose and that we need to employ the services of external contractors to keep us pain-free and comfortable.

By external contractors, I mean things like wrist supports (supposedly needed to protect against the physical rigours of the computer), lumbar support (supposedly needed to protect against the toil of passively sitting in a chair) and memory foam mattresses and orthopaedic cushions (supposedly needed to protect our joints when we sleep). It's commonly thought that such tools of support protect our supposedly vulnerable joints. Please note the heavy emphasis of the word "supposedly" in this paragraph.

Well, I say, "No, a thousand times, no." We've got this entirely the wrong way around. Our bodies become vulnerable *because of* all the cushioned supportive external contractors we use. Contrary to protecting us, the more support and comfort the body receives, the weaker it becomes and the more we are removed from our interaction with gravity.

The more we connect with hard firm surfaces (fig. 19), the more we are forced to put up a fight against gravity. This fight means the body is put under regular challenge and demand. But if the regular demand is not there, the body will preserve energy and switch off the muscles more permanently. As you know by now, muscle weakening will make your movement patterns worse and, over time, substandard movement patterns will lead to more pain.

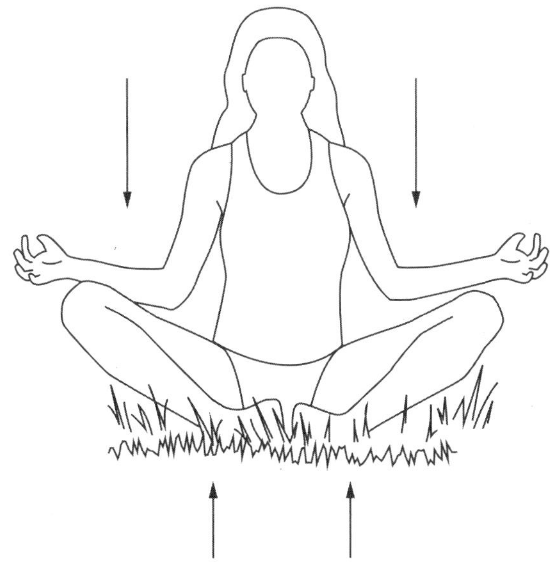

Figure 19: Spending time sitting on a soft surface reduces our fight against gravity, and this weakens our tissues. Spending time on the firm ground (like being outside as shown above) means our body must work harder sandwiched between powerful oppositional forces.

Our bodies don't need support to stay pain-free; they need frequent challenge. For example, if we look at data collected from teenagers in rural Kenya who rarely use chairs with supportive backrests, they tend to have 21 to 41 per cent stronger backs than teenagers from a nearby city who use chairs with supportive backrests.[52] While there is highly likely to be other factors at play, it makes logical sense that the backrests don't help our bodies. They simply allow muscles to give up.

There are, of course, many advancements and benefits that technology and innovation have brought to our modern lives. I, for one, do not want to sleep on the ground or live in a cave. However, my job as a posture therapist is to help you understand why your body hurts. We need to have an awareness of what our bodies evolved to do, and of the mismatch between our primal body and our modern world, to understand why so many of us are living in avoidable musculoskeletal pain.

Sleep well

Next, I want to dig into our sleeping habits a bit further, because I believe our obsession with soft comfortable bedding is one of the leading contributors to muscular weakness, joint imbalance and pain. On top of this, as time has gone on and our sleeping habits have changed, the space between us and the floor has increased and the time we spend on natural firm surfaces has decreased: creating other ramifications for our health, discussed a bit later (page 103).

Let's cast our minds back, once again, to our understanding of what our ancestors did and the resources they had. Our early ancestors would have slept close to, or on, the ground, perhaps padded with some hay or animal skins, or on a rudimentary form of hard bed. It was only when the Egyptians came along, approximately 4,000 to 5,000 years ago, that we raised our beds away from the floor.[53] Before the 1880s, most people could not afford a comfortable mattress,[54] and memory foam was not invented until the mid-1960s.

The support we now get from a soft mattress, like the soft chair, takes away our fight with gravity (fig. 20). And, as explained in Myth 5, constantly working against gravity keeps our bones and muscles dense and strong. Rudimentary bedding will have kept the body muscularly challenged during the night because the fight against gravity won't have been too compromised. All night, with limited padding, our cells would have been dealing with the pressure exerted by gravity pushing down on them and the floor pushing back. This type of challenge keeps us strong because firm surfaces force our bodies to work hard, even when we are resting.

With increased levels of padding in our bedding, we reduce our fight against gravity and we weaken our body. Soft surfaces adapt to the shape of the body, allowing it to soften into the positions we most frequently adopt. Think of jelly melting: that's what happens to our cells and muscles when we spend time sitting and lying on a soft surface. Melting soft muscles cannot hold our bones in the right positions, and this is troublesome if we want to avoid joint pain. We need strong muscles to hold our bones in alignment.

As well as weakening our tissues due to a lack of nocturnal gravitational load, the growing divide between the human body and the natural earth is stripping away the anti-inflammatory benefits to be gained by "earthing" or "grounding" our bare skin on the ground.[55] When we spend time directly connecting with the earth – touching trees, standing in the sea or in a lake, or sleeping on natural ground – we are "plugged in" to the energetic charge of the earth, which is negative.[56] This time spent plugged in helps to reduce inflammation in the atoms of the human body.[57] By being connected to the floor during the night (hay and animal skins are natural conductive materials), our ancestors were naturally and easily reducing inflammation in their body.

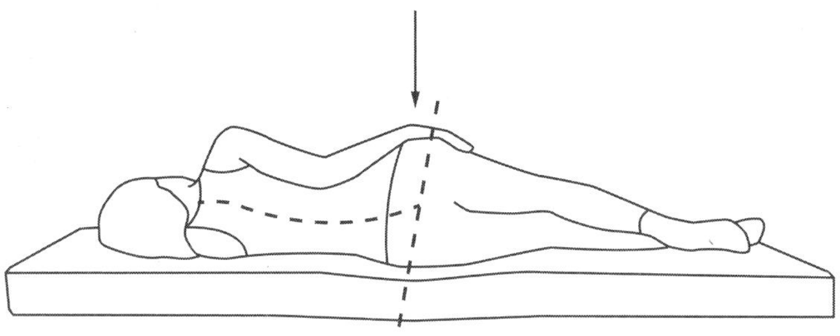

Figure 20: Soft bedding allows our body to melt into the softness, weakening our tissues. Hard surfaces keep the fight against gravity going, even when we are asleep.

Lastly, soft bedding allows us to sleep in positions that, I think, compromise our posture.[58] So many of us (me included if I sleep with pillows) sleep mainly on one side in a curled-up, foetal position with both shoulders rounded forward and elbows bent – all the weight of the body bearing down on one arm. In a soft bed with pillows, I am happy in this position and barely move during the night. However, I often wake up with poor circulation and stiffness in my arm. If I sleep on harder ground – when camping, for example – I can't sleep like this. The ground won't allow me to sleep solely on one side, on one arm. It's simply not comfortable to have the whole weight of my body bearing down on that one arm all night. When I am camping, I naturally sleep more supine on my back for most of the night. Or, when on my side, I have my hands under my head, stretching out the shoulder and armpit. On harder ground, my muscles are staying active, and my joints are interacting with the forces of gravity, even when my brain is not. I always wake up after camping feeling energized and with no stiffness. My body seems to thrive off sleeping on the hard ground, in a more supine position.

When we sleep supine, our hips get the chance to lengthen, relax and release into extension during the night. But if our hips are too tense from lots of daytime sitting, they can't naturally let go. So, for some of us, lying supine can often equate to lower back, pelvic or neck area tension. If you'd like to spend more time sleeping supine, think about using props to change the alignment of certain joints during the night. Things like bolsters or pillows under or between the knees can help the hips and pelvic area release tension, not because they are soft and padded, but because they are modifying your joint positions (fig. 21).

To help me to sleep supine and to generally improve my posture, I don't sleep with pillows. That way, I get the postural benefits of lengthening, relaxing and releasing my neck back over my shoulders and opening up my chest and upper back (fig. 22).[59] Personally, I find that not using pillows encourages me to spend more time sleeping supine, which always leaves me feeling great when I wake up. This is because pillows keep your head cranked at an awkward angle, whichever position you sleep in, and don't allow the head position to reset during the night.

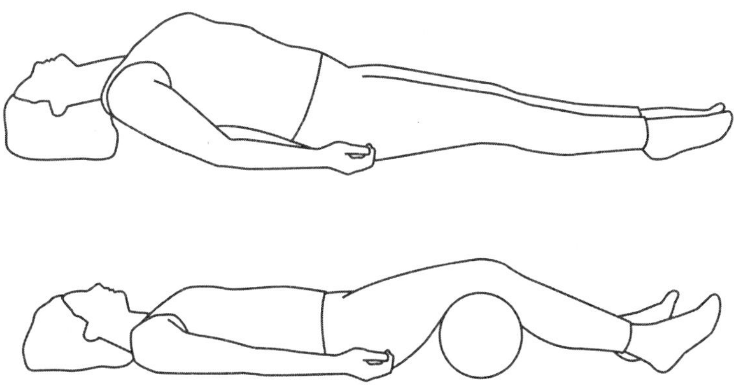

Figure 21: Tense hips while supine versus relaxed hips while supine. Many of us, when lying supine, have an arched lower back, flared ribcage, rounded shoulders and hyperextended neck due to hip tension. Adding a bolster under your knees will allow the hips to relax.

If this information inspires you to change, and I hope it does, go slowly. If your tissues have become used to pillows and you have tension in your body, it's probably not advisable to go cold turkey and get rid of all your pillows straight away. It'll be a process of slowly adapting your tissues to be able to comfortably accommodate a new position. Make the change over several months, during which time gradually use thinner, more dense and fewer pillows.

Some of you may now be thinking, "That's all well and good for you, but if I sleep in any bed other than my own (let alone on the floor when camping), I wake up in all sorts of trouble." Please realize that this is your modern body telling you there is a problem with your muscular function. There is no general biomechanical issue with you sleeping on a hard surface or having less support. You are simply not used to the level of muscular demand being asked of your body.[60]

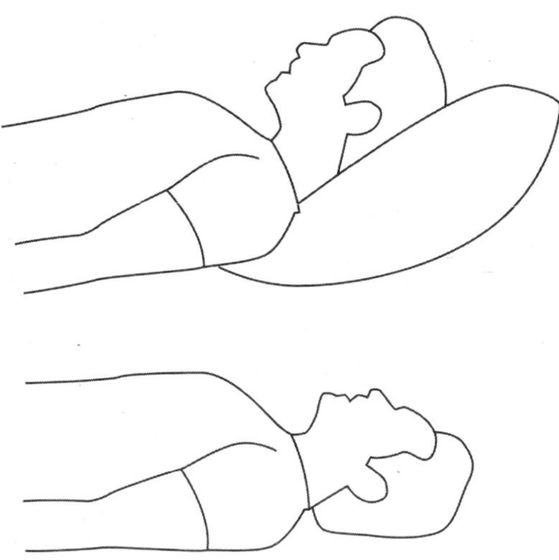

Figure 22: Sleeping with pillows versus sleeping without pillows. The latter allows the head to reposition, the neck and upper back to lengthen and the chest to open.

By doing posture exercises to restore your muscular strength and improve your joint alignment, and also by spending more time on hard surfaces (on the floor and out of a chair during waking hours), you will rebuild your requisite postural strength. Your experience of sleeping without soft bedding and pillows will be dramatically transformed. It just takes some time, work and patience to readapt those weakened cells.

Myth 7: Our feet can't naturally support our bodies Why do we think our feet are so fragile?

Along the same vein, I must speak in more depth about something I feel passionately about: feet and shoes. They are so important I could have written a whole book about them, but really the principle is the same as that explored in the myths above.

The feet contain more than a quarter of the bones in the human body, boast a vast quantity of powerful muscles and joints, and are impeccably designed with a complex arched structure – like an elegant cathedral designed by one of the greatest architects in history. We have elastic Achilles' tendons, evolved specifically for the purpose of running and allowing for propulsion and shock absorption. During our running gait, the Achilles tendon and the arch of our feet work together to return half the force of the body hitting the ground.[61] Our feet are natural, explosive, shock-absorbing power houses.

Additionally, each foot contains about 200,000 nerve receptors to feed our brain important information about the environment and situation we find ourselves in. Our feet and our brain are like best mates who should be in constant communication with each other.[62]

Yet, unfortunately, this exquisite sensory feedback, muscular power and healthy foot structure begin to get stripped away and misshapen from a very early age, from whenever we start to wear modern shoes regularly (fig. 23). The weakened feet of habitually shod populations are not representative of the powerful feet of habitually non-shod populations, and our perspective on what our feet supposedly need can be seriously misinformed and warped.

In my professional experience, one of the quickest and easiest ways to dramatically decrease pain levels across the whole body is by restoring the muscular function back to the toes, arches, ankles, mid-foot and calves by doing the right posture exercises and by transitioning to wearing barefoot or minimalistic footwear. It can, quite literally, be that decades of knee/back/hip/neck pain dissolve overnight when you wake up your feet and start to wear footwear that allows your feet to move as nature intended. Sometimes, if the tissues of the feet are especially weakened and if the structures above the feet are misaligned and bear undue load through the feet (fig. 24), transitioning safely and comfortably into barefoot shoes can take several months. For some of us, it can be a marathon, not a sprint, with a lot of corrective work and patience needed to allow tissues to readapt along the way.

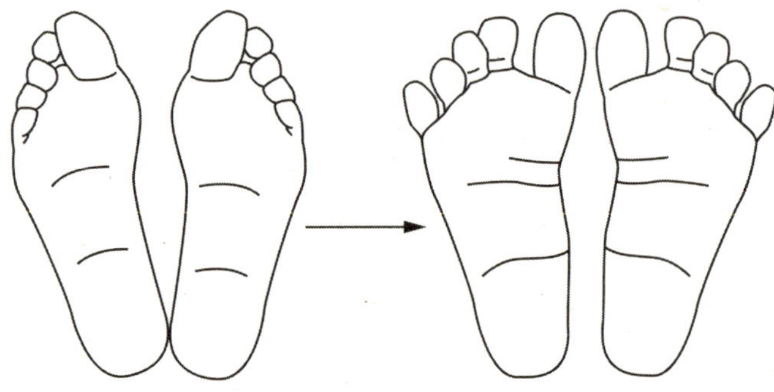

Figure 23: A typical foot shape from wearing shoes versus a natural human foot shape.

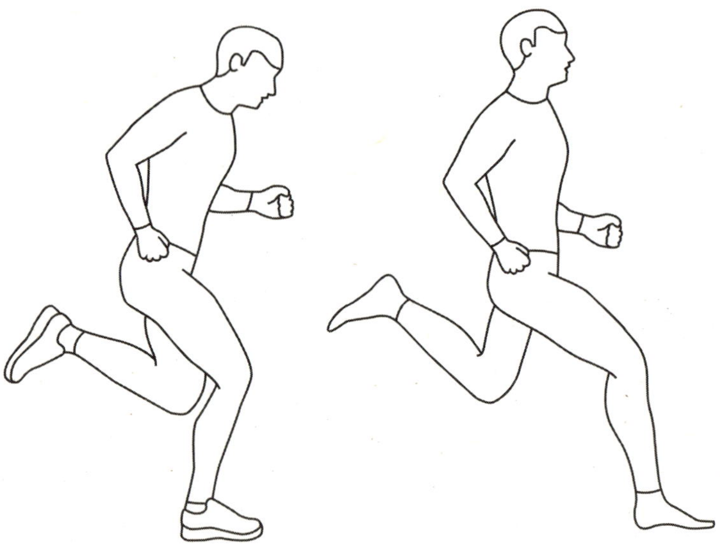

Figure 24: The upper body position impacts the loading of your feet - all the structures above your feet bear an impact on how your feet interact with the ground. In the figure to the left, we see how angled forward the torso is, how rounded the upper back is and how the head is drooping. In comparison, we see how upright the spine and head should be during the running gait.

Let's briefly look back to our early ancestors once again. They would not have worn shoes like we do today. Many people across the world still don't. For most of human history, if shoes or sandals were worn at all, they would have been incredibly simple – created to protect against the elements (as we migrated to colder climes)[63] and from acute damage like cuts and infections. Because all the tissues in the body constantly respond to the load and demand we put on them, when we spend a lot of time outdoors and barefoot, dealing with friction and pressure, we develop thick calluses. These make our skin incredibly tough, like hooves,[64] and deliver a good blood supply to the feet.[65]

Calluses are the body's natural way of making us a keratin-based shoe. If we wear shoes, we don't give our body the demand it needs to create these calluses. Without them, it is hard for us to imagine how easy it is to walk across rough surfaces all day in bare feet. You should see the looks I get when I walk barefoot across gravel. I don't feel anything, because I am used to walking like this and have relatively tough feet (for a shod person), but I get a lot of winces come my way.

By looking at a typical sports shoe from the 1950s and comparing it with the sport sports shoes of today, we can easily see how far shoe technology has come in a short space of time (fig. 25).

It's important to clarify that I am not saying the 1950s sports shoes are optimal (many of them are too narrow, too thick-soled and too stiff), but they are far less complicated than the sport shoes we think we need today. Padding and cushioned support in shoes only came about in the late 19th century with the invention of rubber and, more dramatically, in the 1970s, with the invention of a plastic called EVA (ethylene vinyl acetate), which creates the wobbly foam heel that so many sports shoes now have. This development of shoe technology over the past 100 years or so is not helping us as humans; it's hindering us.

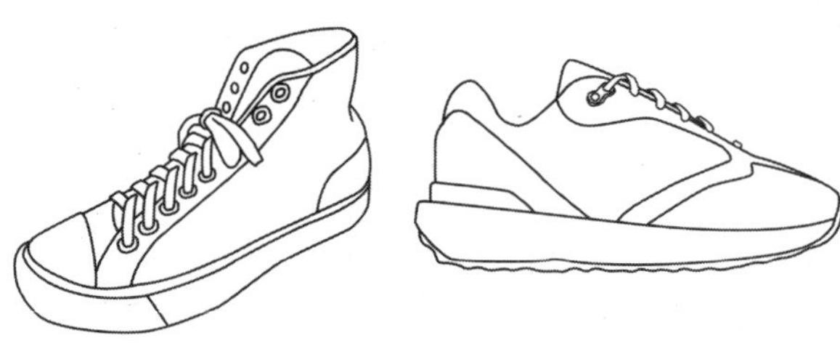

Figure 25: A typical pair of 1950s sports shoes versus a typical more recent sports shoe.

Wearing pointed cushioned slightly heeled shoes is altering your natural human gait cycle. Over time, this change contributes to chronic biomechanical issues, which, eventually, will lead to pain in your body. As with anything that uses support in place of muscular strength, modern shoes switch off our muscles (in this case, in our feet and lower legs) and, as you know, when the muscles become weak, this weakness disrupts the efficiency of the human movement machine and will lead to pain. Wearing gait-altering, toe-deforming and/or wobbly foam "supportive" shoes is okay for a short amount of time or on the odd occasion, but the problem we face is that most of us are wearing these types of shoes most of the time, and perhaps don't realize the damage this is causing.

My intention for every single person I encounter (both professionally and personally) is for them to, at least, hear my viewpoint on supportive shoes and then hopefully, consider transitioning to barefoot shoes. You're encountering me now (!), so once you have read what I have to say, you can make up your own mind about what makes the most sense to you. At this point in my career, I think I have heard every counterargument there is against barefoot shoes, so I hope I can address any concerns you may have in the sections to come.

Before we continue, grab a shoe from your cupboard – one that you wear quite frequently. A trainer/sneaker normally works well to highlight the points I'll make below.

Unlike "normal" shoes, minimalistic/barefoot shoes are a genre of footwear that comprise five main components.

1. A toe box that is wide enough to accommodate a natural human toe spread
2. A sole that is totally flat from back to front (zero drop)
3. No insoles, arch support or padding
4. A sole that is thin and flexible enough to ripple like a wave as the foot strikes/picks up from the ground
5. A design that holds the shoe firmly in place so the toes don't have to grip and so we can pick up our feet properly without shuffling

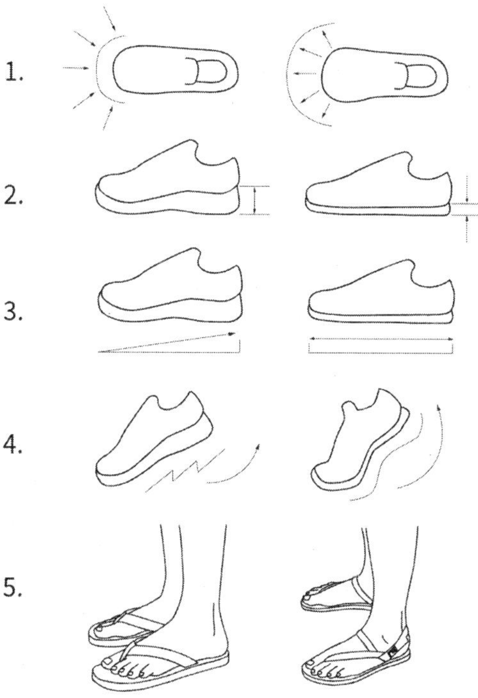

Figure 26: Your minimalistic shoe checklist – wide toe box, totally flat sole, no insoles/arch support, flexible sole and securely attached to the foot.

Now look at the shoe you have selected. I bet it does not pass the checklist (fig. 26). Your everyday footwear needs to meet all the criteria described above if you want to be able to move to your fullest capability and give yourself the best possible chance of living a life in which you're not held back by pain.

But *why* do we need to wear this type of shoe if we want to keep pain-free? It always comes back to considering what the human body has evolved to do. Here are some reasons why modern shoes work against our natural design.

1. Human toes are naturally wide and spread apart like a fan. All you need to do is have a look at a baby's foot (before they wear shoes regularly) and you'll see how the big and fifth toes spread wider than the foot. You may be getting a bit tired of hearing me say this, but every single joint in your body is important and plays its part in keeping you pain-free. Your toes are no different. We need our toes to help stabilize and ground the foot, but they also help us push off through the mid-foot during the gait cycle. If your toes are deformed into a point (by wearing restrictive shoes), your foot cannot be fully stable – and you're also not going to be pushing off through your toes properly. Fundamentally, this alters your human gait pattern.

I thoroughly recommend having a look online and finding some cheap silicon toe separators to wear to start to spread out your stiff toes. Choose a pair that has an equal amount of space between each toe (and that doesn't get narrower toward the end), and then wear them for as long as you can tolerate each day. If your toes are particularly stiff, it may only be a few minutes to start with. But if your toes aren't too stiff, you may find you can wear the separators for a few hours before the muscle burn gets too strong. Slowly increase the time you wear them and your body will adapt. Wearing toe separators is also a great measure to see if the shoes you already have are wide enough in the toe box. If you can't wear toe separators inside your shoes, your shoes aren't human foot shaped.

2. Human feet are not designed to be held in a raised heel. If you wear high-heeled shoes, you know the sweet relief that comes when you take them off at the end of the night. This is because wearing high-heeled shoes angles our feet downward into a range of motion called plantarflexion.

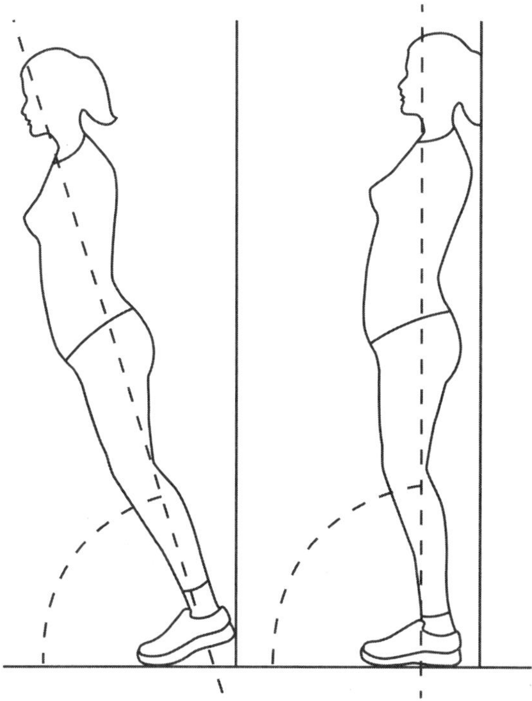

Figure 27: The raised heel of a normal, modern trainer pitches the body forward at the ankle which means the upper body has to pull backward over the ankles to compensate. Over time this creates strain in the lower back and knees.

Plantarflexion is an important range of motion, but it is not one we want to be stuck in. Most normal shoes are heeled, albeit often marginally, and they keep our feet in a perpetual state of plantarflexion. Having our feet angled downward without the ability to counteract the plantarflexion with full dorsiflexion (pulling backward the top of the foot toward the shin) is tiring because it pitches our body forward on a constant diagonal. We then either overload the front of the feet/toes or we pull our upper body back (out of this diagonal), thus overloading the lower back and creating strain (fig. 27). You cannot escape one of these two compensations when you wear even marginally heeled shoes.

Constant plantarflexion also keeps the calves and hamstrings in a state of overwork and tension. As the calves and hamstrings become more dysfunctional, this prevents the hips and pelvis from moving correctly and creates a cascade effect of movement issues throughout the whole body. We need flat soles on our shoes so our feet can plantarflex/dorsiflex equally to maintain balance in our movement patterns, from bottom to top.

3. Human feet need hard work to stay strong. Like all the other tissues in the body, our feet do not need cushioning – they need work. This is for several reasons. Cushioning takes away our body's productive and natural fight against gravity, which strengthens it (when aligned and functional). In the same way our soft bedding and squishy sofa allow our muscles to melt into a puddle, so do our cushioned shoes (fig. 28).

Cushioning in shoes allows the muscles to switch off and become dysfunctional. Why would the foot muscles wake up when they don't have to? Conversely, having no cushioning in the shoe forces the foot to work hard through necessity. The more the muscles of the feet can work and operate powerfully, the more the other joints of the body are protected.

Cushioned footwear also means we are wobbling around on an unstable foundation, like constantly walking around on the surface of a trampoline (fig. 29). Unstable foundations create unstable structures that will suffer wear and tear further upstream. With this instability, is it any wonder so many of us roll on and hurt our ankles?

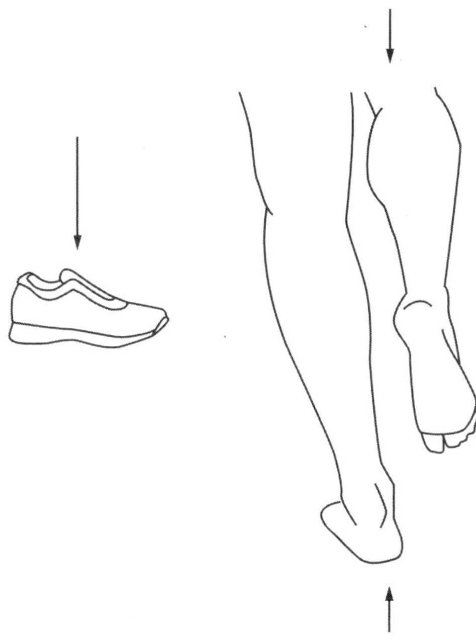

Figure 28: Our idea of normal sports shoes interrupts our fight against gravity and switches the muscles off (which eventually overloads our joints elsewhere). Moving around barefoot keeps the functional fight against gravity going.

Feet are meant to strike firm ground, and our contact with firm ground means our feet can push off with precision and power. If our feet land on an unstable surface, such as shoe padding, this wobble ricochets through the body into all the joints. The ankles rock side to side (and potentially lead to sprains), the knees wiggle and overload and the whole upper body has to brace itself (read, stiffen) to prevent us from falling over. Also, if we support the arches of the feet with an insole-type contraption, not only do we switch off the muscles in the arch of our feet, but we also prevent our mid-foot from properly flattening into pronation and lifting into supination as we walk, which is part of the natural gait cycle.

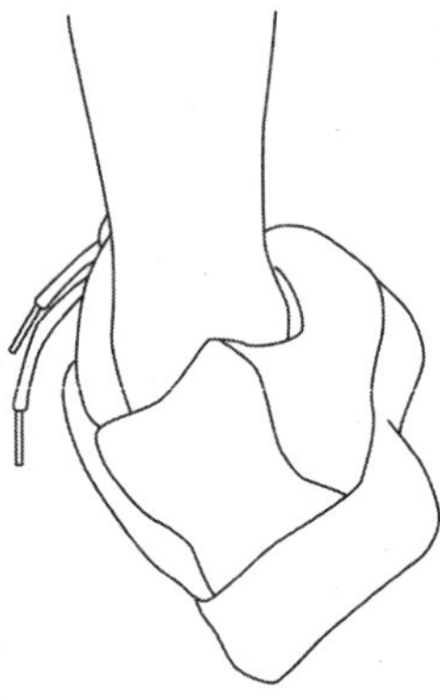

Figure 29: Wearing wobbly shoes means we are moving around on an unstable base.

4. Human feet need to articulate like a wave when they strike the ground. Thin soles allow each section of the foot to move individually, as it should. We can think of our walking gait as like a boat rocking forward and backward on the sea, with some side to side movement, too. When we walk functionally (barefoot or in minimalistic shoes that don't alter the natural human gait pattern), we touch the floor with our heel and our foot rolls onto the outside edge into supination (lifted arch position), then the mid-foot rolls down into pronation (flattened arch position) and then we land through the ball of the foot to push off powerfully from the big toe joint.

When barefoot we run differently, with a much lighter, more mindful, more delicate gait pattern, during which the foot connects to the ground at the mid-foot, not the heel.[66]

Cushioned trainers encourage and allow a heel strike. If we are wearing thick stiff soles, with no movement to them, our feet do not receive all the nuanced movement of rocking our ankles, feet and toes through the gait cycle. Stiff soles encourage us to land heavily in a heel strike (fig. 30), and push off at the toe end of the shoe, with little movement or shock absorption through the mid-foot. This pattern feeds into stiffness and dysfunction, particularly in the mid-foot. Think of thick stiff soles as turning your feet into trotters, making the whole length of your foot (heel, mid-foot, ball and toes) hit the ground almost at the same time. Such soles limit the ability of the joints of the feet to articulate. The more your feet are stiff like trotters, the less stability and balance you will have in your feet, and the more the other joints in your body will have to brace and compensate. The more the other joints brace and compensate? The more pain they are in.

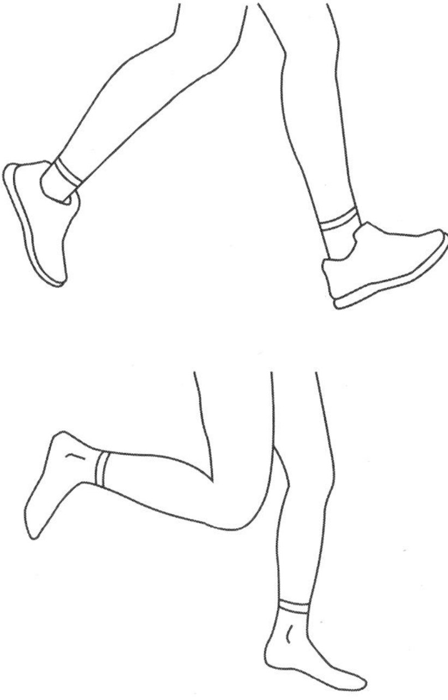

Figure 30: Padding in shoes alters our gait and allows us to heel strike, which is not the way we would run barefoot.

5. Human toes aren't supposed to grip shoes in place. I'm afraid your Birkenstocks, sliders and flip-flops aren't safe from my barefoot scrutiny. Because they are not firmly attached to your feet, these types of shoes make you shuffle while you walk. You can't pick up your feet, lift your knees and swing your legs properly through hip flexion and extension when your body is also having to navigate holding an unsecured shoe on your foot. If you spend a lot of time shuffling, you will eventually lose the muscular function required to allow you to walk properly.

Additionally, shoes without secure fastenings often create a toe grip. The toes are forced away from their actual job of stabilizing the foot and pushing off from the ground, and are, instead, distracted and waylaid into holding the shoe in place. If you knew how the exhaustion of your gripping toes feeds a line of tension through the rest of your body, you might be less inclined to wear unsecured shoes. Please don't be fooled into thinking that Birkenstocks, sliders or flip-flops are barefoot shoes just because the sole is flat(ish) and they are open-toed. They come with their own host of movement problems.

Counterarguments against barefoot shoes

I mentioned earlier that I think I've heard all the counterarguments there are against barefoot shoes, and they normally boil down to slight variations on the five points below. Hopefully, I can help alleviate any scepticism you may have about barefoot shoes and get you curious about changing your body and your movement by changing your shoes.

1. If we are supposed to wear minimalistic shoes, why don't top athletes wear them? That's easy: a top athlete's priority probably isn't being pain-free and functional; their priority is winning the race. I admit, you will most likely run a lot faster in cushioned heeled shoes that propel you forward like a spring. But comparing running in cushioned trainers with running in barefoot shoes is like comparing driving a car and riding a pushbike: one is faster than the other but not necessarily better.

Running in minimalistic shoes requires the muscles in your body to work hard to propel you forward as you push off and then deal with shock absorption as you land. You've got no outside help to assist you, so you're relying on your muscular strength, function and power alone. To run in barefoot shoes requires a great deal of whole body function. It is a real reflection of the true nature of how functional your movement patterns are.

Let's take a look at bodybuilding to explain my point. There are bodybuilding competitions where it is accepted that competitors use steroids to enhance their performance, and there are natural bodybuilding competitions where it is not acceptable to use steroids. They are not comparable competitions. The bodybuilders who have taken steroids most likely will lift heavier weights and have more muscle definition. However, there's a cost to using performance-enhancing drugs; steroids may help you win a competition, but they are disruptive to your health. So, it depends on what is more important to you: winning or staying healthy?

The same is true for cushioned shoes (the performance enhancer). They may help you run faster than you would if you relied solely on your muscles, but they prevent you from moving naturally and they create an unstable base that offsets your entire structure and switches off your foot muscles. So, the long-term cost will most likely be pain somewhere in your body (not necessarily in your feet). As an example of pain showing up somewhere you may not expect, look back at figure 27. It reveals how raised heels pitch you forward on a diagonal and the upper body compensates to pull backward over the heels to balance the human structure. As the upper body fights back against the force of the pitching forward at the ankles, it puts strain on the lower back and the knees.

Finally, look up Abebe Bikila. Some people are *so* functional in their movement patterns they can win a marathon barefoot!

2. The environment has changed so much – our ancestors didn't have to deal with concrete or tarmac. Admittedly, hundreds of thousands of years ago, there was no concrete. But there was the sun-drenched African savannah, stony tracks and large rocks that humans would have spent a great deal of time navigating. Many entirely natural surfaces are, in fact, dense and unforgiving, just like concrete. We evolved out of these environments and our bodies will therefore have adapted to cope barefoot with natural hard surfaces.

Early forms of concrete were first used around 9,000 years ago (much earlier than many of us realize), and ancient civilizations like the Romans and Greeks built stone roads. These certainly won't have been forgiving surfaces and we certainly didn't have cushioned shoes back then.

We evolved to regularly walk or run over a great deal of different surfaces of different textures and gradients, and our feet are not designed to walk or run on flat surfaces all the time. However, I don't believe flat surfaces (concrete or tarmac) are a problem in themselves, provided the rest of our movement profile is challenged enough to balance out the uniformity of the flat surface. Uniformity is the problem here, because uniform surfaces do not take muscles and joints through a wide enough range of movement to keep them fully functional.

To prove this point, here's a little testimony. I am someone who does not enjoy running and hasn't run in years. I do spend a lot of time walking in minimalistic footwear on different gradients and surfaces, and I invest heavily in maintaining my mobility across my body. Recently (at the time of writing), I ran a two-hour half-marathon in minimalistic barefoot sandals. I had no joint pain or muscular tension at any point in my training, during or after the half marathon itself.

Despite my personal lack of love for running, I agree with the sentiment that humans are "born to run" because there are adaptations in our physiology that suggest this.[67] Additionally, it's highly probable that our endurance in "persistence hunting" animals over the course of a day (with much stopping, starting, walking and waiting allowing us to frequently cool off while the animals overheat with exhaustion) has allowed us to dominate as a species on Earth.[68] However, knowing what I know about our innate desire to conserve energy, I don't think our early ancestors would have thought going for a run every morning was a good use of their time or energy.

By this reasoning, I agree that earlier generations would not have frequently run long distances on hard surfaces – because they wouldn't have frequently run long distances, non-stop, at all. Running long distances regularly, non-stop, for fun or exercise is a new phenomenon and not one for which the human body evolved. There may have been some people, like messengers, who had to make long distance runs, but they would have been in the minority.

If we agree that humans weren't made to run long distances frequently, especially not on concrete or tarmac, then why don't we reconsider how often and how long we are running for? Would it not be better to do a different form of exercise rather than to wear a cushioned shoe that alters our biomechanics to unnaturally load our joints?

I know this suggestion will make the blood boil of athletes and running club members across the world, but hear me out. I'm writing this book to help you understand how evolutionary and modern-day environmental mismatches cause us pain, and I'm trying to point you in the direction of changes you can make to create an environment and movement profile that is more suited to your primal body. You can make of this information what you will.

In short, if your goal is to stay pain-free, I encourage you to spend less time running on concrete or tarmac, more time running over different gradients and surfaces (because of how great this is for our movement profile and ranges of motion) and more time investing in improving your mobility outside of your running – so your body becomes more resilient. Also, I encourage you to find time to safely transition to barefoot shoes, so you can sense feedback from your body and realize how much better it feels.

To clarify my stance here: I believe we are born to run in the pursuit of food or in self- or community defence. I think we are amazingly capable and strong across all surfaces, provided we keep our joints and muscles healthy through a varied and balanced movement profile and do not wear shoes that alter our movement patterns and our body's interaction with gravity. I believe that running (with a balanced musculoskeletal system and an efficient running gait) is great for the health of our joints and the strength of our bones. I think running can absolutely form part of a healthy balanced movement profile and that our physiological adaptations for running would suggest it is good for us to run. However, I do not believe we are supposed to wear cushioned shoes to run long distances, non-stop, almost every day, without other varied movements that help to maintain joint and muscle health.

3. I need insoles because I have flat feet. I posit that you have flat feet, in part, because you have worn cushioned footwear for most of your life. You can change your flat feet, but they will need the right muscular stimulus. That's because flat feet are a symptom of a movement problem, not the root cause of the problem.

The arches of our feet begin to develop when we are about three years old, and they often don't stop developing until we are around ten years old.[69] So, we need to give children's bodies the chance to develop their foot arches at a natural pace. Worryingly, some children have insoles put in their shoes when their feet are still developing and when nearly all feet are flat. This early use of insoles creates the thing they are supposed to help with: weak flat feet. Because insoles are a form of support, they allow the muscles to melt and switch off, meaning that many children don't ever get the chance to develop their arches. The long-term use of insoles makes the foot flatter and unable to cope when the insole isn't being used.

Flat feet are a sign that muscles all over the body aren't working properly. The good news is that, with the right posture exercises, you can change your flat feet entirely. With more propulsion and power through the toes, feet and ankles, you can begin to lift the arches of the feet. It's not only this improved foot function that will change the feet though. Flat feet are normally also a sign of weakness and instability in the hip and pelvic area (fig. 31). Consequently, we also need to engage our hips, thighs and glutes to prevent our knees from rolling in, and to stop these collapsed knees from also creating a collapse in the feet.[70]

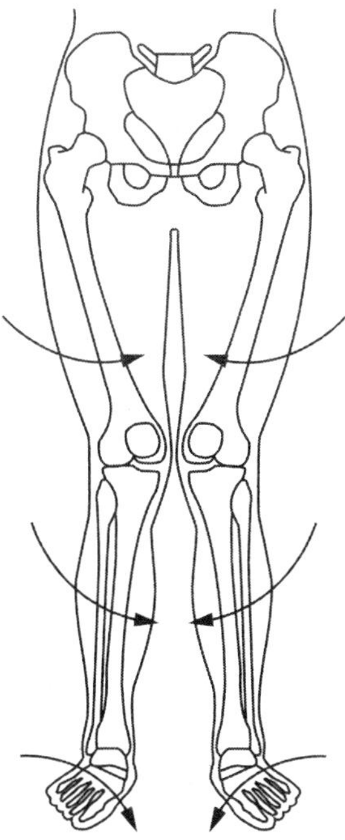

Figure 31: When the muscles of the inner and outer hips are dysfunctional, the bones of the legs are not supported properly. This instability often presents as an internally rotated position of the femur and knee and a collapsed position of the inner foot. Change the inner and outer hips and you'd lift this entire chain.

4. If cushioned shoes are an issue, why do companies still make so many? You want my short answer? Money. Call me a conspiracy theorist, but I don't believe that multibillion-dollar businesses have our best interests at heart. I think shoe manufacturers know exactly what they are doing. I believe they know that the shoes they are peddling are creating weakness and pain in their customer's bodies. In my opinion, the motivation for shoe companies is dependency, because the more weakness and pain someone suffers and the more they are told they need cushioned shoes, the more reliant that person becomes on cushioned footwear. Healthy feet cost less to maintain, and so don't make as much money for shoe manufacturers. I believe it to be that simple.

5. I get pain when I go barefoot but not when I wear cushioned soles and insoles. Your personal response to going barefoot is another way your body reflects your whole body muscular function and posture back to you.

If your muscles and joints struggle when you go barefoot or wear minimalistic footwear, this is your body trying to tell you that something needs to change. You need to pay attention to how the muscles all over your body are working (this is not just a foot issue). When we mask our symptoms of foot pain (or possibly knee, hip or back pain) with padding (cushioned shoes and insoles), it's like taking a painkiller. Padding allows us to quieten the all-important pain messages we need to listen and respond to, and by doing so we allow our body to continue substandard movement patterns for longer. The longer we get away with moving poorly, the more our joints will suffer. The cushioned shoes aren't stopping your joints from wearing away; they are simply preventing you from hearing crucial feedback.

If you wear cushioned shoes to hide from pain – and especially if you do this and continue with higher intensity activities (like running) – the problem will insidiously get worse, but you just won't feel it anymore. At some point, the biomechanical issues that your body is trying to alert you to will shift elsewhere.

If your movement patterns are substandard, padded shoes will numb you to your body's feedback, whereas barefoot shoes will hold up a mirror to the problem. Being barefoot or wearing minimalistic shoes is not causing your pain; it is simply allowing you to hear a message from your body and I believe it's important to listen to this.

TEST YOUR POSTURE

Do your feet work?
In-line Position posture test

For those of you currently wedded to the idea that your feet need the support of external technology (rather than from functioning muscles in your feet), here's a posture test. This is a posture test for weak feet, but also one of my favourite exercises for strengthening weak feet.

We are going to test to see if your feet are currently capable of performing one of their key functions: holding your body upright and stable.

1. You'll need to be barefoot. Ideally, find a straight line on the floor. This could be the line of a tile or the edge of a floorboard. You are going to create an invisible tightrope and see if your feet can balance you on the tightrope.
2. Set your feet up one behind the other (fig. 32) on the line. Note how the line goes through the centre of the second/third toes and through the centre of the foot and bottom of the heel. Relax your toes and make sure there's no scrunching. Pin into your big toe joints on the balls of your feet. They are your anchor.
3. Relax your arms by your side. No clenched fists, no hands on hips and no hands out in front of you in "prayer position".
4. Your knees should be straight, but not locked backward into hyperextension.
5. Your weight should be balanced through each foot, and make sure you're not favouring one leg over the other.
6. When you look down, your pelvis should be balanced. Make sure one hip isn't twisting forward in front of the other.
7. Now, hold this position for three minutes and then swap to the other side, with the other foot in front. Keep breathing and relaxing your belly throughout.

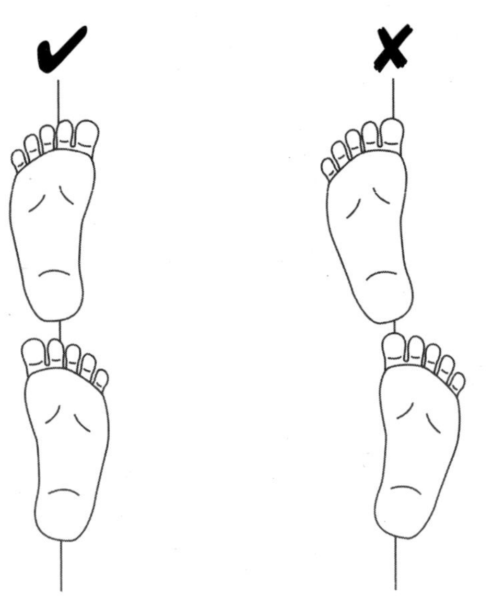

Figure 32: When doing this test, be very careful on the alignment of the toes. The arms need to be relaxed by the side and bodyweight centred inbetween both feet. When you look down at your pelvis, make sure one hip is not further forward than the other.

What happens when you do this test? Are your arms flailing about wildly? Are you struggling to maintain your balance in this position? Are your ankles and calves burning? Is your rear hip on fire? If so, great, you have learned that your feet are currently not very good at supporting the rest of your body. Maybe this is why you feel you need support from your shoes – because you are not getting it from your feet.

Being able to hold this position easily and calmly means your feet are good at some ranges of motion called pronation and supination (fig. 33). Think of a boat bobbing sideways on water; this is a bit like pronation and supination. If the feet are functional in these ranges of motion, they are used to stabilizing the rocking motion. The feet may wobble a bit, but the rest of the chain (knees, hips, pelvis, spine, shoulders and head) is not really impacted or unstable. The feet can stabilize themselves.

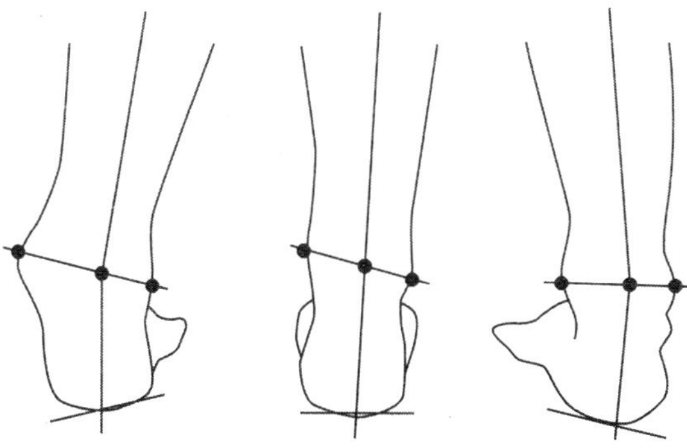

Figure 33: Pronation is the inward rocking of the foot (flattening of the arch) and supination is the outwards rocking of the foot (lifting of the arch). Our feet need both ranges of motion in order to hold themselves in 'neutral' while at rest.

If your feet are not functional at moving through pronation and supination, they do not have the muscular strength to also keep the rest of the joints in the body stable. With dysfunctional feet, the unstable wobble at the feet also tugs at the whole structure upstream, causing instability and imbalance – as you may be experiencing in this posture test.

The more we work to strengthen our capacity to move functionally through pronation, supination and the other ranges of motion available to our feet, the sturdier our feet become and the more stable and relaxed all the other joints in the body are, too.

Padded supportive shoes take away the demand for this rocking sideways range of motion, so we become increasingly dysfunctional in pronation and supination.

As we become more incapable of performing these types of movements ourselves, we become more dependent on the cushioning that likely caused the dysfunction in the first place.

A body held upright by strong feet is a much sturdier body to live in and one that suffers a lot less instability further up. As you know now, instability causes wear and tear in the joints and tension in overworking muscles.

So, we don't need cushioning in our shoes; we need foot strength. If you found this test difficult, repeat it as an exercise every day, and soon enough you'll become a lot more stable when you do it. The feet work hard and the rear hip burns as it "talks" to the feet holding it steady. You may notice aches and pains elsewhere in your body magically reduce, too.

TAKEAWAYS

1. To move pain-free, we want to keep our movement profile as varied as possible.
2. We evolved to be movement generalists, not movement specialists. We cannot do one form of exercise and give our joints and muscles everything they need, especially not in our generally sedentary environment.
3. We need to prioritize restoring and retaining mobility across the body.
4. The human body's constant fight between gravity and the ground is one of the natural ways we stay strong and resilient.
5. Many modern conveniences, such as soft beds and soft chairs, interrupt our natural ongoing fight with gravity. This constant fight strengthens our bones and muscles.

If we cushion, support and protect our bodies too much, over time, it weakens our tissues.

6. When our tissues are weak, they cannot hold our joints together efficiently, causing pain.
7. It's a great idea to begin to reduce the height of the pillows you have, so you can restore your head and neck position through the night.
8. Cushioned heeled shoes interrupt the proper development of our feet, our fight with gravity and how all our joints hold themselves. In turn, these interruptions affect how much pain we get.
9. If spending time barefoot or in minimalistic shoes causes you pain, keep your padded shoes on, but start working on your posture to restore your movement patterns. Keep testing to see how it feels to spend short amounts of time barefoot. Your body will tell you when it's ready.
10. Toe separators will help prepare your feet for more barefoot time, and they will also help you move better.
11. Transitioning pain-free to minimalistic footwear can take a fair amount of time if the feet are particularly weak or if the structures above the feet are positioned in such a way to overload the feet.
12. Getting your body functional enough to spend time barefoot or in minimalistic footwear is a wonderful sign of posture progress. If you can get to the point where barefoot time is no longer painful, it means you have improved your strength, your alignment and your mobility.
13. Humans are born to run, but not in the way most of us do now.

Conclusion

I hope I have already encouraged you to think a little differently about posture, and I hope you are ready and keen to start making some changes. In part 4, I'm going to provide some practical ideas and exercises, but first I would love you to hear me out on why I think posture is even more important and all-encompassing than we currently realize.

Part 3 "My Hunches" describes some of my theories that are based on logic, supposition, research and anecdotal evidence. I am not stating concrete truths, but I am pitching ideas for consideration. I trust that you will find my views, at the very least, compelling.

PART THREE
MY HUNCHES

YOUR HOUSE

Movement helps all the systems of our body function better

Movement reduces our risk of developing most chronic lifestyle diseases, lessens many symptoms of those same diseases, boosts our chances of living longer, improves our mental health and so much more. This is such common knowledge that it needs little explanation. My hunches are not about convincing you that you need to move. They are here to get you thinking about how the *position* of your body as a whole and the *position* of your individual joints within your body – rather than movement itself – impacts all the systems in your body: how the position of your ribcage impacts your ability to breathe; how the position of your shoulders impacts the circulation in your hands; how the position of your hips impacts your digestion; how the position of your spine impacts your neurological function; and how the position of your pelvis can make pregnancy and giving birth more uncomfortable and difficult.

To illustrate this, I want you to view your posture like a house, the house you live in. Think of your muscles, bones, ligaments, fascia and tendons – your musculoskeletal system – as being the foundations, the bricks and mortar of your house. Within the house, you also have plumbing, electrical wiring, lighting, internal walls, a heating system, a roof, carpets, curtains and furnishings. In my analogy, these various things represent your cardiovascular, neurological, respiratory, lymphatic, digestive, excretory, reproductive, endocrine and urinary systems. I believe that the structural integrity of the house itself will bear a huge influence on the longevity, function and efficiency of everything inside it (fig. 34).

If the foundations of the house start to subside and cracks begin to appear in the walls, over time this loss of structural integrity will impact how the wallpaper stays on the wall, how efficiently the plumbing system can operate, whether roof tiles start to slip off the roof and whether or not damp creeps in.

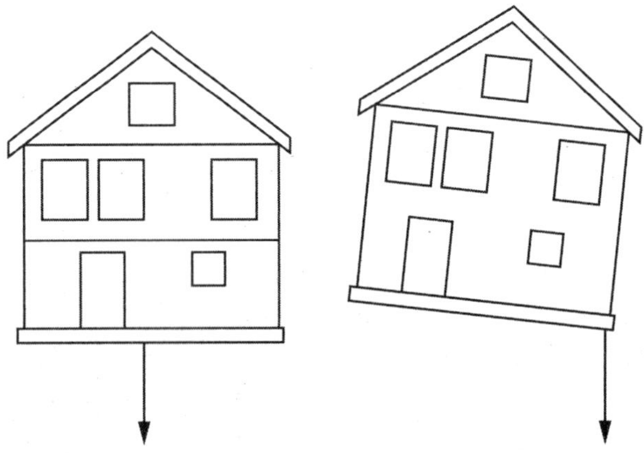

Figure 34: The house on the left represents balanced functional alignment of the musculoskeletal system. The house on the right represents the typical imbalanced posture that many of us will be living within – all the time. Long term, what happens to the things inside this structurally unstable house?

The interconnectedness of all the systems in the body is not a new idea. Much of Eastern medicine is based on the premise that balance is needed across all the systems of the body to maintain holistic health, and several Western doctors have echoed this sentiment. In 1895, Dr Edmund Shaftesbury claimed, "Posture that caused the chest to slump was the particular villain, for then the organs could not operate independently and the action of heart, kidneys and liver was impeded."[71] And, in 1943, orthopaedist Walter

> Posture that caused the chest to slump was the particular villain.

Truslow posited that balanced posture would lessen the strain on the structures within the body and help to maintain vital organ function and efficiency.[72] Sadly, it seems, the people who made these observations were not taken particularly seriously. The wisdom that I believe was held in these statements was never truly explored on a larger scale and so didn't fully benefit current Western medicine and attitudes.

It is my belief that the modern medical system is still missing a trick, and that many of us are still not seeing how neurological, digestive, hormonal, cardiovascular and other seemingly unrelated health issues are, in part at least, being impacted by the dysfunctional postural structure in which they reside. Of course, there are many factors that contribute to the health of the systems of our body, but the position of the joints is a crucial piece of the puzzle that is most probably not getting enough consideration. If we work to improve our posture, are we also – finally – digging into the root cause of many different types of currently unexplainable conditions and illnesses? I believe so.

In part 3, I am going to hypothesize the connection between our posture and five of the systems of the human body: respiratory, cardiovascular, nervous, digestive and reproductive. I believe that posture impacts all the systems of the body, but I chose these five examples because I feel they are the simplest to grasp.

You may notice that the sections in part 3 seem to overlap. This highlights the fact that everything in the body is connected.

CHAPTER 9
POSTURE AND THE RESPIRATORY SYSTEM

My hunch: Your posture impacts your breathing (and vice versa)

Let's kick this off by hearing from one of my clients. If you are someone who is plagued with breathing difficulties, her testimony may give you hope that the answer you seek may be simpler than you think.

> *"I had already raised my breathing to a better level using mouth tape for well over a year but, when starting posture, I did so with an eye toward alleviating my left leg sciatica pain and reducing both my forward head posture and rounded shoulders.*
>
> *Unexpectedly, about one month into the routines, I suddenly noticed that it was October and I was not, and had not been, using my inhaler for my asthma.*
>
> *That month had historically been the very worst for me. Having developed asthma at age 32 (I am twice that age plus some now!), when it was at its worst I used the inhaler three times per day, every day. The reduction in use six months into committed posture work is such that I use the inhaler once every two weeks or so – barely at all.*

It has been such a good feeling to have improved posture with the bonus of improved breathing.

And, by the way, the goals of less pain and improved postural elements have happened! I owe both the inspiration and, of course, the instruction to Ellie. Her combination of methods, based on her experience, has proven to be a game-changer for my entire body – full stop!"

Martia

The relationship between posture and breathing is quite straightforward. But first, let's take a quick look at what the respiratory process involves. Every cell in our body needs oxygen to function, because oxygen breaks down glucose into energy and this is how we feed our cells. Our respiratory system is how we get oxygen into our body. Ideally, we should breathe in and out through the nose. Nasal breathing means that the incoming air is filtered and warmed by the nasal passage, as it travels down the trachea into the lungs and into the diaphragm, which then expands to continue a slow controlled inhalation of air deep into the torso (fig. 35). Breathing through the nose also stimulates the release of nitric oxide into our body. This is a super important part of the respiratory process. Among a host of other benefits, nitric oxide lowers blood pressure, aids our immune system function and helps our lungs to absorb more oxygen.[73] As the air hits the lungs, the lungs feed the newly oxygenated blood into the blood vessels of the cardiovascular system and into the rest of the cells in the body.

Then, there is a short amount of time in which we should hold the inhaled breath, allowing a build-up of carbon dioxide. Our body needs a build-up of carbon dioxide during the short breath hold because that build-up creates a more powerful and efficient inhale of oxygen afterwards. Think of the difference in pressure, during a breath hold, between the inside and the outside of the body, helping to more powerfully draw in the oxygen on the inhale. After this, the diaphragm slowly contracts to gently push the carbon dioxide-laden air back out of the nose. The cycle then begins again.

I like to think of the diaphragmatic inhale as stimulating and waking up the body, and the diaphragmatic exhale as relaxing and calming the body. The exhale and inhale are equally important when it comes to functional respiration (and the functional use of the muscles of respiration), but the exhale is crucial for making sure we are releasing stress from our body.

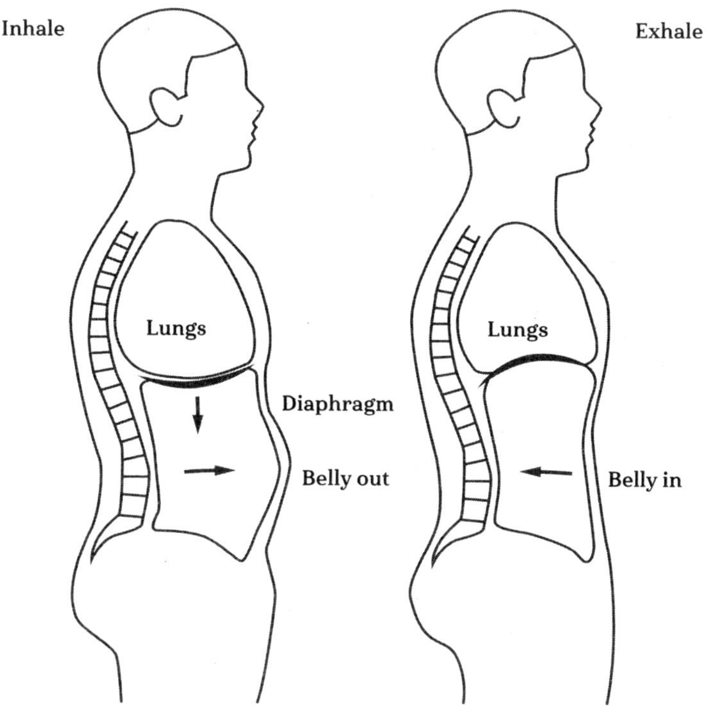

Figure 35: The diaphragm is an expansive muscle located across the bottom of the lungs and ribcage. It moves up and down and outward and inward with the inhale and exhale of the breath.

LET THE BELLY GO

I have explored diaphragmatic function in greater detail above (pages 138–139), but I'll share an important point here. You will not catch me teaching my students to pull in their belly during posture exercises. If you are habitually gripping your abdominals, you are not "protecting your lower back" nor "strengthening your core"; you are creating tension and dysfunction. Abdominal gripping stops you from breathing properly, it stiffens your torso and spine, and it allows the muscles of the hips and pelvis to switch off (because the abdominals are compensating). By breathing properly and by moving your torso frequently in all sorts of directions, you will strengthen your lower back and core. You cannot create optimal posture by trying to hold yourself unnaturally. So, let your belly go and get your diaphragm moving.

Upper body positioning

Is your posture causing long-term compression in your lungs, ribcage and diaphragm?

In chapter 3, I mentioned that I don't like to use the words "good" or "bad" in relation to posture (pages 38–39), but I am going to use them here, briefly, because those terms help illustrate the point I'd like to make. When you think of good posture, you picture someone standing or sitting tall with an open chest and shoulder position. When you think of bad posture, you imagine someone standing or sitting slumped over with a closed chest and shoulder position (fig. 36).

What do you think is happening to all the systems and organs inside the body if you stand or sit in a slumped position? I believe they are being compressed and functionally impeded, including the respiratory system. Try for yourself: slump like the figure on the right (above) and try and breathe through your nose for a few breaths into your diaphragm. Then, sit up a bit straighter and try again. Do you notice a difference?

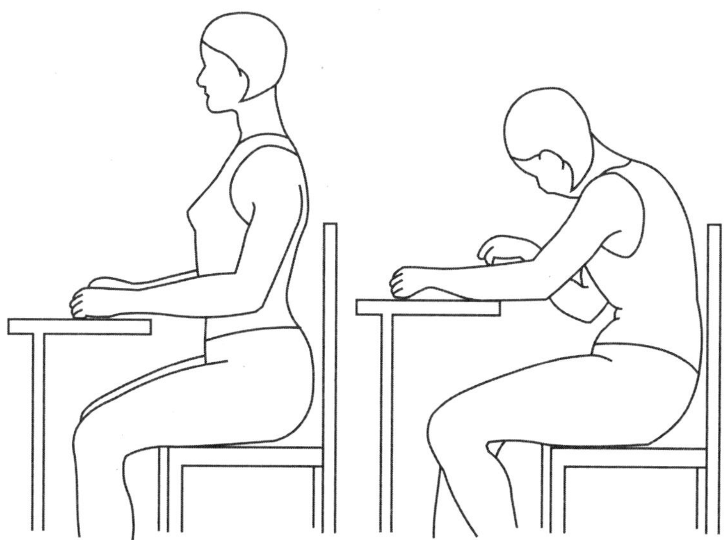

Figure 36: An open chest position versus a compressed chest position. Imagine the position of the lungs (and everything else inside the torso) in both people.

Because the tissues in your body are constantly adapting to the load and demand put on them, if you spend a lot of time in a compressed position while sitting down and become stiff in this type of posture, you'll get to a point where your body cannot decompress itself, even when you stand back up. This is muscular dysfunction at play and it is a prime example of getting "stuck" in a posture. At a certain point, the respiratory system may become constantly compressed in all postures and movements.

As you will have noticed when you tried to breathe in a slumped position, when your body slumps forward and your torso area is compressed, you impede the ability of the diaphragm to move functionally. And being able to move the diaphragm is critical to facilitating functional breathing.

In my opinion, the diaphragm is one of the most important postural muscles in the body. It has many roles to play in maintaining good health, including – but not limited to – helping to pull the lungs and chest into a more expanded position to allow for more oxygen absorption, improving blood flow, maintaining body temperature and circulation, helping us retain a springy pelvic floor, maintaining our torso area posture, keeping our hips relaxed, and stimulating the vagus nerve (a long nerve that sends information to and from internal organs and the brain) that passes through the diaphragm. The last is one example of how the systems in our body interconnect, as both the respiratory and nervous systems directly interact in the diaphragm (which is also part of the musculoskeletal system and cardiovascular system).

Is your posture affecting your stress levels?

The vagus nerve connects the brain with most organs in the body. It is a crucial part of activating the parasympathetic nervous system, the side of your nervous system that calms you down and allows your internal systems to "rest and digest". If the vagus nerve is regularly stimulated (for example, through moving the diaphragm, laughing, yawning, chanting or humming), it helps to bring us out of a stressed "fight or flight" response. The opposite is also true. If we aren't stimulating the vagus nerve enough, we are not sufficiently teaching our nervous system that we are safe. If we do not feel safe regularly, we are more likely to remain stressed. This stress then feeds into all the other organs of the body, via the vagus nerve and other channels of communication, contributing to chronic overload and ultimately organ malfunction.[74] In chapter 11, we will consider the importance of your posture and your nervous system more generally, but here, I want to look specifically at the respirational relationship between the diaphragm and the vagus nerve.

We have established that the movement of the diaphragm is part of what stimulates the vagus nerve and keeps feeding back to the brain the message, "You are safe, let's stay calm". If we spend a long time in a position in which the diaphragm cannot move, we are helping to keep our bodies in a fight or flight state.[75] My hunch is that our sedentary stuck posture is a crucial factor in what could be keeping us chronically stressed.

Chronic mouth breathing = chronic stress Noses are for breathing; mouths are for eating

> *"When I started posture training, my goal was less neck and knee pain. Now, in addition to being pain-free, I am stronger, more sure-footed and breathe better than I have in my entire life.*
>
> *It's stunning how much easier it is to improve dysfunctional breathing habits when your body is properly aligned. Along with better breathing, my anxiety has lessened, as have my allergy symptoms.*
>
> *My body is no longer the thing that just carries around my brain. I move well and have gained an awareness of how all the parts work together.*
>
> *I feel more confident too.*
>
> *The posture transformation has been more than I expected, in the very best way."*
>
> *Jen*

In moments of physical stress, such as running away from a tiger, we can recruit our mouth to help out our nose to get more emergency air into our lungs. However, please note the use of the word "moments". We are not designed, as humans, to habitually mouth breathe, and yet many of us do. When we habitually mouth breathe, the impact is far-reaching and quite dire. Here are just a few side-effects: allergies, hay fever, poor circulation, asthma, sinusitis, chronic fatigue, impaired brain function, immune system dysfunction and anxiety – all exacerbated or even caused by mouth breathing.[76] If there are so many downsides, why are so many of us mouth breathing?

In my opinion, we mouth breathe, by and large, as a stress response or as a forced postural response, and these two factors play off one another and exacerbate the problem. When the body is panicked or stressed, it will perceive the need for more oxygen to convert into more energy. Therefore, the desire to mouth breathe will be activated. Posturally, if we are sitting down and slumping while simultaneously becoming stressed – not able to use our diaphragm to help calm us down and improve our air flow – we will be more likely to recruit the mouth to breathe. Without the diaphragm moving properly, nose breathing will probably make us feel like we aren't drawing in enough air, so we will rely on the mouth even more. A simple scenario: if you are sat at work reading annoying emails, you may well be mouth breathing for two reasons: the physical necessity of the compressed chest and diaphragm position, and as a physiological response to ongoing stress.

The more stressed and sedentary we are, the more likely we are to chronically mouth breathe – and mouth breathing then becomes a habit we struggle to break. We are familiar with the phrase "use it or lose it" being applied to our muscles or brain, but the nose is the same. If we don't use our nose to breathe, we will lose the ability to use our nose to breathe,[77] because the regular inhalation of air through the nose helps to keep our sinuses, nasal cavities and throat cavity unblocked. Thus, once we are in a vicious cycle of physically not being able to breathe through the nose, we end up being further trapped in a cycle of mouth breathing.

Luckily, making improvements works both ways. Improve your posture and you'll improve your breathing patterns, because better posture results in more space for the respiratory system to operate. Improve your breathing and you'll improve your posture, because better breathing patterns result in more movement of the ribcage and our posture, therefore, changes. In fact, dysfunction of the diaphragm and poor breathing are two of the main contributors to a forward head posture. When the respiratory system doesn't have the proper support of the diaphragm, the head learns to seek out a sub-optimal position where it can best draw in oxygen.

Improving your posture by doing corrective exercises helps to restore the mechanics of respiration by improving the functional movement of the diaphragm and ribcage. Better movement of the ribcage can not only help to open the hips, chest and shoulders and pull the head back over the shoulders, but also lift us out of a state of chronic stress. Through our posture exercises, we can train our respiratory system to work more functionally and harmoniously (creating a cascade effect of other benefits). We can learn to naturally unblock our nasal passageways and immediately calm our nervous system by activating the vagus nerve through diaphragm stimulation. The time you spend practising how to breathe properly – aka the time you allocate to your posture exercises – will gently translate into a virtuous cycle: you will naturally be able to move your diaphragm more throughout the day, which will help to keep you calmer, but the time spent practising will also reduce your stress levels, so you can deal with your daily life in a less reactive way.

POSTURE EXERCISE

Unblock your nose
Nose Clearing Breath

When I speak about the importance of nasal breathing, one of the things I glean is that many of us already know we should be breathing through the nose. However, often our nose and sinuses are so congested that we physically can't do nasal breathing, despite our best efforts.

If this is you (or even if it isn't), you may want to try this exercise, taken from Patrick McKeown of The Buteyko Method.[78]

Please do not attempt this posture test (which involves creating an air hunger to change the biochemistry of your blood to help clear your airways) if you are pregnant, over the age of 60, have high or low blood pressure, strong anxiety, panic disorder or cardiovascular issues, or if you have any serious medical conditions. I'm not saying you can't learn to unblock your nose naturally, but please consult a breathwork practitioner first.

Note: When you get to instruction 3, make sure you do not hold your breath for so long that you gasp after letting go of your nose. The next inhale after letting go of your nose needs to be relaxed and quiet, so don't overdo the breath hold until you understand your limits.

1. Take a few breaths in and out through your nose to get an idea of how it feels and how congested you are. Make a note of any differences between nostrils.
2. Take a low slow nasal breath deep into your diaphragm. When you reach the limit of your comfortable inhale, gently but fully exhale all the air out of your nose. Close your eyes and pinch your nose closed using your thumb

and index finger. If you're extremely congested, pinch your nose straightaway – rather than inhaling and exhaling first.

3. Continue to hold your nose shut, and slowly nod your head up and down for about five to ten nods.
4. Once you have completed your nods, release your nose and – before you breathe out – take another relaxed deep inhale in through your nose. Then breathe out. Give yourself 30 to 60 seconds rest and go again. Repeat this process five times – so six times in total.

Do you notice a difference in how congested your nose feels? I hope so! If you do, I suggest you practise this exercise frequently. As you become more able to hold your breath in an increasingly relaxed way, extend the number of nods you do. The more you can build up your tolerance to air hunger, the more efficient the exchange between oxygen and carbon dioxide becomes.

If you don't feel any different, don't worry! There are many other breathwork exercises you can try, and there will be one that works for you. You just need to keep exploring. At first, you may need to focus a bit more on diaphragmatic movement, rather than creating air hunger.

Another thing you may wish to consider – to encourage nasal breathing – is to wear mouth tape at night.[79] While the idea may be a little daunting at first, wearing mouth tape is one of the easiest ways to reintroduce the habit of nose breathing. It's been an absolute game-changer for me, my husband, so many people I work with and several high-profile athletes.[80] My bedroom is now blissfully quiet, we wake up more refreshed and without a dry mouth, we sleep better and we also naturally nose breath so much more readily throughout the day. Wearing mouth tape is truly transformative and perfectly safe. The mouth tape I use goes around (not over) the mouth and gently encourages (not clamps) it shut. You can still open and close your mouth throughout the night if you need to.*

TAKEAWAYS

1. Our posture and our respiratory system are intrinsically linked.
2. We cannot have good movement patterns if we don't have good breathing patterns.
3. We need our diaphragm to be able to move in and out fluidly for many reasons, including to stimulate our vagus nerve. This nerve helps put our body in a state of "rest and digest", and so calms us down and allows our organs to repair themselves.
4. Gripping the belly or "tightening the core" is problematic for our breathing patterns and posture, and I never give this cue in my classes. Strengthening your core functionally does not happen from artificially tensing your muscles.
5. Being sat in a chair compresses the lungs and prohibits the diaphragm from moving. This can lead to more mouth breathing.
6. The more we mouth breath, the less we filter and warm the air coming into our body. This compromises our immune system, creates inflammation and keeps us stressed.
7. You can learn to naturally unblock your nose and clear your sinuses through posture and breathwork exercises.
8. Using mouth tape is an easy way to learn to nose breathe without having to think about it.

* In part 4, I will share various recommendations to help you improve and understand your posture, including a recommendation for mouth tape.

CHAPTER 10

POSTURE AND THE CARDIOVASCULAR SYSTEM

My hunch: Your posture impacts your blood flow

The cardiovascular system involves pumping the blood around the whole body through a network of arteries, veins and capillaries: the blood vessels. This network delivers the newly oxygenated blood from the heart and brings the deoxygenated blood back to the heart. Blood helps to fuel every system within the body, including the movement of muscles. However, movement also synergistically helps to fuel the cardiovascular system, because movement helps to flush the blood and lymph (fluid that flows through the lymphatic system) back toward the heart.

The relationship between the cardiovascular system and movement is symbiotic. In a body starved of movement, the heart must compensate and work harder than intended to move blood around – because the movement half of the relationship is not pulling its weight.[81] I believe there are quite far-reaching negative health consequences to having a habitually compensating heart in a sedentary body.

Many of us already know that regular movement is critical for the health of our heart and our cardiovascular system. The challenges that movement brings keep the heart strong and stops the residual build-up of plaque from clogging the blood vessels, helping to prevent the blood vessels themselves from stiffening.[82] But my hunch is that the impact of our posture on the cardiovascular system runs deeper than this.

Looking at the images of the cardiovascular system and the musculoskeletal system in figure 37, I think it's obvious that the two systems are interrelated. The blood vessels weave themselves in and out of all our muscles and bones. I believe the positioning – posture – of the muscles and bones impacts the function of the cardiovascular system. So what happens to the blood vessels in a body where the muscles and bones are not being held in the most efficient anatomical position? Their function becomes impeded.

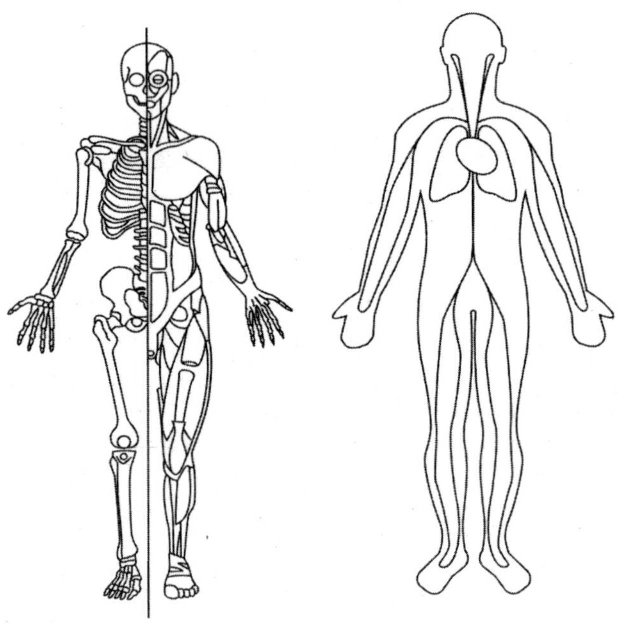

Figure 37: The musculoskeletal system and the cardiovascular system intertwine throughout the body because the muscles are fed by the cardiovascular system and because deoxygenated blood is transported back to the heart via movement.

Circulation
It's not just about gloves and socks

You can see in figure 37 how many channels of the cardiovascular system are housed around the lower legs/feet and the lower arms/hands. When we complain of circulation issues, so often it is the hands and feet that seem to suffer most. Clearly, the hands and feet are further away from the heart than other body parts and so the blood has further to travel. In terms of blood supply – in a body that is not moving enough or that is under a lot of stress – the hands and feet will be less of a priority than the vital organs. Our body is good at making do with what it has and making sure that the critical bits of us – needed for our survival – are served first.

I believe there are more posture-specific reasons why we may suffer bad circulation, beyond the fact that many of us simply aren't moving enough to make the blood swirl around nicely to keep us warm. Let's consider the posture that many of us sit in for hours daily: the typical slumped over the desk position, with rounded shoulders and crossed legs (fig. 38).

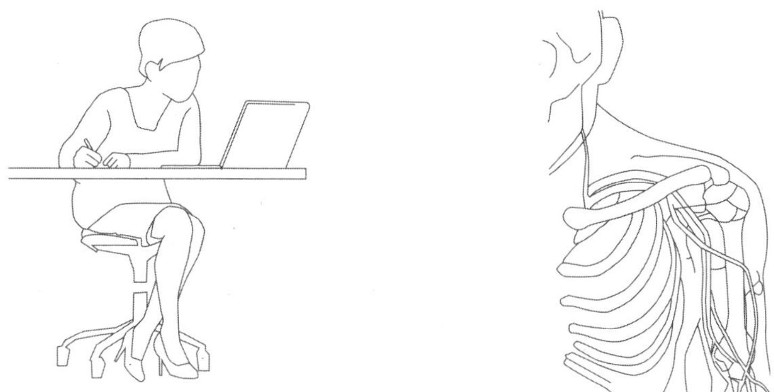

Figure 38: Slumped shoulders will compress the blood vessels that feed down into the arm.

How do you think the compression in the front of the chest (caused by the slumped shoulders) impacts the blood vessels that feed down into the arm? The collarbone and other bones in that area will start to close in on themselves and this will insert pressure on the blood vessels, impacting blood flow. Think of the blood vessels as being a water pipe, and pressure on the blood vessels from the joints turning off the tap. This principle explains why you may wake up with a dead arm in the morning if you have slept on one side all night (compressed nerves also contribute to this).

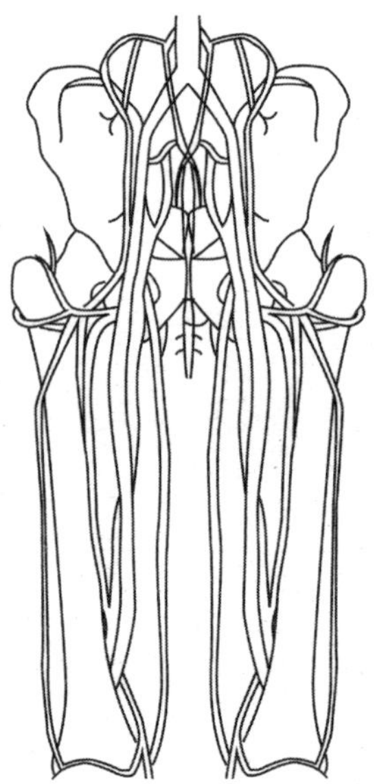

Figure 39: A web of blood vessels resides around the lumbar vertebrae, pelvis and hips, feeding down into our feet (fig. 38). Crossed legs will impede these blood vessels.

The same goes for our legs (fig. 39). If we habitually sit on a chair in hip flexion, I can't help but think that the blood "tap" feeding down into our feet will be compressed and switched off. I believe poor circulation to the feet directly stems from a lack of movement through the feet and compression in the hip and pelvic area. Not only that, the same postures that compress the blood vessels in the front of the chest and the hip area will also compress the nerves that run through those areas to the limbs, causing numbness, tingling and coldness in the hands and feet.

As we know, muscles that are not stimulated often enough will eventually stiffen up and become dysfunctional. When our muscles become stiff and locked in certain postures, the bones become stuck in that posture, too. This means that a temporary circulation issue that presented itself only in certain postures – such as lying on your side in bed and having a dead arm in the morning – may become more permanent. If the body cannot unstick itself from the postures causing the blood vessels to compress, I believe a more problematic circulation issue will begin to emerge and feed into symptoms like Raynaud's syndrome (in which blood vessels to the extremities narrow and restrict blood flow)* and chilblains (inflammation caused by exposure to cold and damp). As the circulation of the blood becomes more permanently impeded, areas of pooling and stagnation will begin to form.

Bulging and varicose veins
A symptom of stagnation

> *"I'm in my third trimester of my second pregnancy and I recently noticed that I was starting to have some heavy pelvic tension and an increase in my varicose veins at the top of my legs. I was then diagnosed with vulvar varicosities.*
>
> *The tension was becoming unbearable, to the point on some days that standing up was causing so much pain and my varicose veins were bulging.*

* Circulation issues are also exacerbated by dysfunctional breathing patterns. Learning to create a greater tolerance to air hunger is a really good way to improve circulation in your body.

I did one of my posture routines and it completely blew me away as, when I stood up after doing that class, I was instantly met with pelvic relief, and I also noticed my veins looked less swollen.

I repeated the same class every day for two weeks and, since doing so, my symptoms have massively reduced.

I can only think that how my posture has changed during pregnancy has affected my circulation, and the posture exercises [Ellie] provides help my body to be able to function well again. So thank you, I feel so grateful to always have posture exercises to keep me out of pain.

No matter how hard I try, posture is the ONLY thing that I have found where I am almost able to 'fix' myself."

Angi

I believe varicose veins are a symptom of a lack of movement and undue long-term pressure on the blood vessels. Varicose veins are commonly seen in the lower extremities, and they appear when the blood pools in a particular area and isn't being flushed away correctly. The work of the heart pushes blood away from the centre of the body, but if we are sedentary and we are not moving our feet and legs enough to stimulate the blood's return to the heart, the blood stagnates downstream and can't complete its cycle. Not only that, but our modern footwear prevents our feet from moving in the way they should, causing deformation of the toes, stiffening of the mid-foot and impacted mobility of the ankles. Without the functional movement of our feet, ankles and calves, we struggle to flush the blood (and lymph) back upstream. So, even if we are trying to be less sedentary, our choice of footwear may be getting in the way of our cardiovascular health by impeding functional foot and ankle movement.

A general lack of movement doesn't adequately explain why we get differences in our veins from one side to the other. For example, some of us get a lot more pooling of blood in one leg over the other. This is where imbalanced posture comes in. The appearance of your veins is a useful clue to where the problem lies: they tend to show you where your blood is pooling and, therefore, where there is not enough movement happening. For example, if you have varicose veins in one calf but not the other, it indicates that there is less movement and more muscular tension occurring around that calf (and maybe you'll notice your circulation is worse in that leg, too). As a right-handed person, I have a bulging vein in my right arm and much worse circulation in my right hand than my left. But, remember, you need to stretch out more than just the area of the body that offers the visible clue. The whole body needs to be worked and balanced holistically as a unit, so that restricted muscles and veins can be released.

If you notice parts of your body where the blood vessels seem crooked, a different colour or more prominent, it is highly likely that this is where your muscular restriction and postural imbalances are prohibiting efficient blood flow. With the correct exercises, I believe you can get that blood pumping nicely again and reduce the bulging in your veins.

Using posture to lower blood pressure

One of the best tools to reduce stress

Some of the modern world's most serious and most common health issues, such as heart disease, hypertension and heart attacks, relate to blood pressure and the cardiovascular system.[83] Of course, blood pressure can become elevated for several reasons, but one of the causes of blood pressure dysfunction is the impact and inflammation that comes from long-term chronic stress.[84] When we experience a lot of pressure and tension in our daily life and we live in a near-constant state of low-level fight or flight, I believe that higher intensity exercise is likely to increase our cortisol (stress hormone) levels and make us feel more stressed out. Although we need movement to stay happy and healthy, and high-intensity exercise absolutely has its place in a regulated nervous system, I think we need to understand that the exercise we choose influences the mental state we are in.

One of the most accessible ways to reduce our stress levels and, therefore, potentially reduce the risk of stress-related blood pressure and cardiovascular issues is to use our physiology to our advantage and move in a low-impact gentle way, with a real focus on the breath. Working on your posture can help you do this. In a stressful situation, gentle movement (combined with a breathwork practice) is a great companion, because it helps to pull us out of our wired thinking brain and back into our more primal grounded brain – but without elevating our cortisol levels and exhausting us too much. Witness a mammal have a stressful experience, and you'll notice they often shake themselves afterwards. This is them intuitively moving the stress out of their system using something called a neurogenic tremor, so the trauma doesn't get stuck inside their body.[85] We are mammals and we should also be doing this.

The exercise we choose influences the mental state we are in.

I believe that the more we move, the more we shift our energetic state and stop stress from lingering in the body. But, if reducing stress is the goal, we need to remember to move in a compassionate mindful way. For example, a CrossFit class, may not be what your body needs right now; you may benefit more from down-regulation breathwork (twice the length of the exhale to the inhale) and more grounded gentle exercise such as yoga or tai chi. Exercise can raise or calm your mental state. Both effects are valuable, but be sure to choose wisely to suit where your nervous system is at.

TAKEAWAYS

1. Our blood vessels feed our muscles, and so are interlinked and intertwined with them.
2. The position of our muscles impacts the position of our blood vessels. Our bones and muscles may compress our blood vessels (and nerves).
3. If you have circulation issues, you probably have postural and breathing issues.
4. I believe that varicose and bulging veins are caused by tension and a lack of movement in the impacted area.
5. We can use exercise to relax us, calm our nervous system and lower our blood pressure. Be sure you are doing the right type of exercise.

CHAPTER 11
POSTURE AND THE NERVOUS SYSTEM

My hunch: Your posture impacts your nervous system (and vice versa)

"After an accident aggravated and exposed Tarlov cyst disease (which causes debilitating sacral and buttock nerve pain plus numbness and a whole host of other undesirable outcomes), I found myself confined to bed, as all movement intensified pain to the point of only being able to lie still on a heat pad to relieve it. Gentle chiropractic helped, but the adjustment didn't hold for long.

Divine intervention led me to Pain Free,[86] *which explained how untangling tight muscles and fascia was key to becoming pain-free. I thought maybe untwisting my spine would relieve the pressure on the nerve roots and get me out of pain.*

I carefully tried the passive 'static back' pose and could hardly believe something so simple could have such a profound effect. Even as I lay there, my pain decreased. I was instantly converted from that moment and listened to podcast after podcast to learn more.*

* I share this posture exercise with you in chapter 16.

Since then, I have done posture work daily and, even though I am still limited in what exercises I'm able to do, my quality of life has improved dramatically. A surprising side-effect of undoing years of accumulated stress and tension is that my body is changing shape for the better as well. I'm not healed by any means, but I feel I'm on the right path."

Yvette

The interrelationship between posture and the nervous system is a topic that, for me, warrants a whole book. I'll try to cover the basics for you in a single chapter!

In my opinion, the impact of our posture on our nervous system is broadly two-fold. First, I believe imbalanced posture contributes to, or even causes, many neurological (relating to the nervous system) conditions, some of which we don't currently fully understand. Second, I think imbalanced posture contributes to a constant state of fight or flight in our nervous system – and, vice versa, being trapped in a constant fight or flight state contributes to imbalanced posture.

Like the cardiovascular system, the nervous system weaves an enmeshed path through the musculoskeletal system. In fact, if you look at images of the two systems, you'd be forgiven for mistaking them for one another (fig. 40).

In a nutshell, the human nervous system comprises the central nervous system, which is made up of the brain and the spinal cord. The peripheral nervous system connects the central nervous system to the other parts of our body, such as our limbs and organs. The brain creates a message (pick up the phone), the spinal cord delivers the message, and the peripheral nervous system acts out the message (hand picks up the phone). This works the other way around, too. The peripheral nervous system can create a message that will travel via the spinal cord to the brain. For example, if you put your hand on something hot, your nerves will fire a warning signal to the brain via the spinal cord. The brain recognizes the danger and instructs you to remove your hand. So, the nervous system is a busy two-way street between the brain and the rest of the body. To work optimally, it is dependent on the ability of the spinal cord to deliver accurate and efficient messages between the central nervous system and peripheral nervous system.

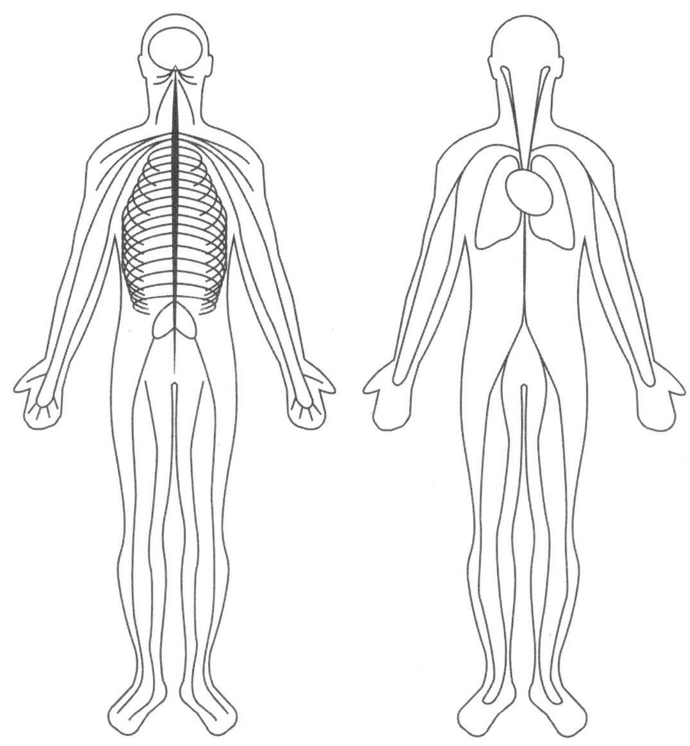

Figure 40: Nervous system (left) and cardiovascular system (right).

It is important to note that the nervous system is responsible for creating movement in the muscles, which subsequently create movement in the bones. Some of us are already aware that our nervous and musculoskeletal systems are intrinsically linked function-wise, but I believe there is more of a relationship to uncover than we currently realize.

Spinal alignment and neurological conditions

The spinal cord is the motorway of the brain, and it needs structural integrity

One of the most common neurological symptoms I come across in my work is sciatica. This occurs when the sciatic nerve, located around the pelvis and lower back, becomes impinged and sends nerve shockwaves down through and into the lower leg. The reason the nerve becomes impinged is due to imbalanced muscles in the pelvic area pulling the bones out of place, and these bones cause compression on the nerve. It's incredibly simple to address sciatica through posture exercises that balance the pelvis and lumbar region.

> *"Working with Ellie on my posture, has truly transformed my experience with sciatic pain.*
>
> *Before I started doing her programme, I struggled with constant discomfort in my lower back and legs, and I had noticed a persistent hip hike that made things worse. Ellie's approach to improving my posture and addressing the imbalances has made all the difference.*
>
> *With her expertise, I've experienced significant relief from my sciatica, and my posture, including the alignment of my hips, has improved drastically. I feel more balanced, confident and pain-free thanks to her guidance. I'm incredibly grateful for the positive changes Ellie has helped me achieve!"*
>
> *Amrita*

If sciatica, a neurological symptom, is caused by pelvic and spinal misalignment, how many other neurological conditions are caused by the same issue? I believe there are many.

In figure 41, you can see the extremely close positional relationship between the vertebrae of the spine and the spinal cord of the nervous system. The spinal cord (and many other nerves stemming from it) is held in place by the support provided by the vertebrae of the musculoskeletal system.

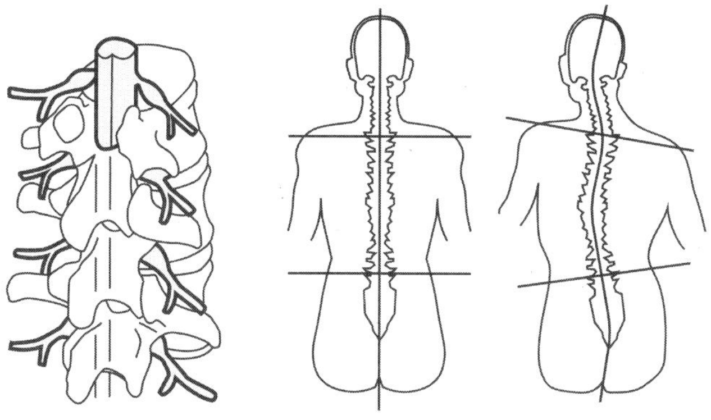

Figure 41: The spinal cord's location relative to vertebrae of the spine. Functional spinal alignment versus a common example imbalanced spinal alignment (see how a wallet in a back pocket or crossed leg could do this over time?)

Figure 41 gives you a wider perspective of the entire "home" that the spinal cord needs to operate within. The vertebrae of the spine are designed to stack neatly in a vertical column, situated on top of a balanced pelvis, with a balanced ribcage, balanced shoulders and balanced head. I believe a spine that holds itself like this – feeling free, mobile and upright – serves as an efficient courier for the nervous system.

You may have heard of a spinal condition called scoliosis. In our sedentary and mentally stressful modern world, spines that hold themselves in perfect alignment – over the course of a lifetime – are rare. Scoliosis is a condition in which the vertebrae of the spine are not being held in optimal postural alignment. In figure 41, you can see there is rotation and lateral deviation, or sideways twisting, of the vertebrae in the spine on the right. As is the nature of posture, when one part of us loses alignment, other parts lose alignment, too. Everything in the body is connected, and if you have scoliosis in one part of your spine, the rest of the spine must compensate and adapt, causing more scoliosis through your entire spine. The condition will impact how your shoulder blades sit and how your arms hang, as well as your head position and your pelvic position.

While some of us are medically diagnosed with scoliosis, it is my belief that many of us will develop a level of scoliosis during our lifetime but may never get a diagnosis. You may not, therefore, know you have scoliosis. To check: reach your hand around to your spine and feel every vertebra you can from the top of your neck all the way down to your pelvis. Even if you are new to this posture stuff, I am confident you will be able to decipher if certain vertebrae are misaligned, are more protruding against your skin or are hidden behind other vertebrae. If you detect any of these, you probably have scoliosis in your spine.

Some of us are born with scoliosis (for example, if we are born with too many vertebrae in the spine), but I believe that even sometimes a diagnosis of scoliosis at a very young age can have a postural cause. For example, if a baby suffers a traumatic birth, their breathing patterns may be dysfunctional or their pelvis may be twisted from the start; or if a baby spends a lot of time sitting in a baby bouncer, this may intercept the natural development of their postural muscles and impact the alignment of their bones.

Scoliosis can also develop over the years for a number of reasons: non-diaphragmatic breathing patterns will impact the alignment of the ribcage, sitting cross legged and slumped forward in a hunched position for long periods in a desk chair will hike up one side of the pelvis and rotate the ribcage, and lying on your side in bed may cause your spine to become twisted. Just like any other part of the musculoskeletal system, the spine reacts to the demand put on it.

A whole system disruption. If the main delivery channel (spinal cord) of our nervous system is disrupted by our spinal alignment, what is going to happen to the function of the nervous system? I would hazard a guess that it will be disrupted, too. Here's an analogy: someone posts a letter in a letterbox and there is a hardworking postman on the other end willing to deliver the letter. But if the sorting office is in disarray, is that letter going to arrive punctually? No. Apply this same logic to your nervous system. Your brain, your limbs and your organs may be functioning well enough, but if the middle man – the spinal cord – is not able to do its job, I believe problems will arise. As ever, all parts of the body need to operate well for the whole system to run efficiently.

This is not a groundbreaking revelation, but I firmly believe more research needs to be done to investigate the correlation between poor spinal alignment and many neurological disorders. Another hunch is that a dysfunctional nervous system caused by poor spinal alignment will have a significantly larger reach than just neurological disorders. The nervous system is hugely involved in the operations of all the systems in our body, so if the nervous system is dysfunctional, surely none of the other systems are working optimally?

Within the scope of my experience as a posture therapist, it makes perfect sense to me that improving the alignment of the spine through posture exercises would improve the position of the spinal cord. In turn, this would allow the nervous system to communicate more efficiently across all the systems of the body, thus improving the symptoms of neurological (and potentially many other) conditions.

Imbalanced posture = chronic stress (and vice versa)

Are you stressed because of your posture? Or is your posture stuck because you're stressed?

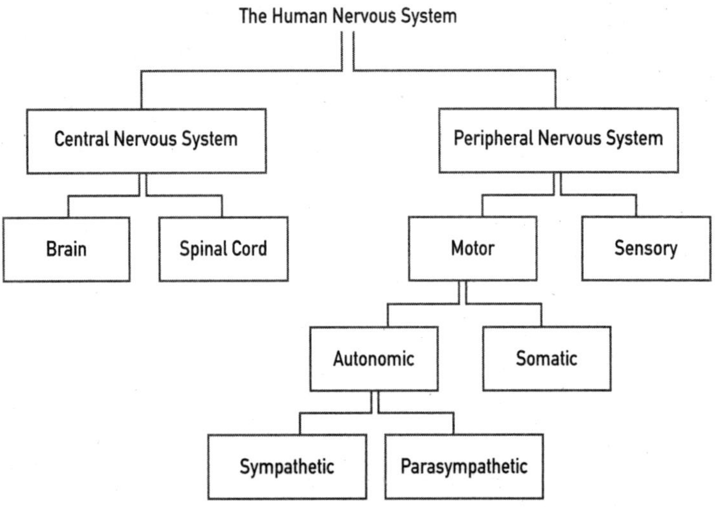

Figure 42: A map of the human nervous system.

We're going to look at stress again, but first I need to expand a little more on the various branches within our nervous system network. The peripheral nervous system has several subdivisions within it (fig. 42). One of these subdivisions is the autonomic nervous system, which drives the things we control subconsciously (such as our heart rate), and the other is the somatic nervous system, which drives the things we control consciously (such as kicking a football).

Within the autonomic nervous system are another two subdivisions: the parasympathetic nervous system and the sympathetic nervous system. The parasympathetic nervous system is our state of "rest and digest", when our organs can repair themselves and the body is peaceful. The sympathetic nervous system is our state of "fight or flight", when our body is on physiological alert and, therefore, not able to think about relaxing and repairing.

Modern life often involves a low-level near-constant state of chronic stress: bleeping phones, never-ending to-do lists, bills to pay, and juggling work and family life. It can be hard to find the regular state of rest and digest that our body so desperately needs every day to replenish itself.

On top of these chronic daily stressors, most of us are also living in a state of poor postural alignment. Due to our sedentary lifestyles, the "house" our body lives in is collapsing around us, and this is impacting the functioning of all the body's systems, creating more stress. Our misaligned posture is not helping our stress; it's adding another problem to the pile.

We can flip this narrative on its head. Yes, imbalanced posture causes more stress, but more stress also causes imbalanced posture. If we are super stressed, we are likely to find ourselves – consciously or unconsciously – holding a lot of tension in our body. I'm sure you can relate to receiving an unwelcome email and noticing your shoulders shoot up to your ears. This is the outside world bearing an impact on your posture.

As I mentioned earlier, I believe humans – just like other mammals – are designed to shake tension out of the body after a stressful encounter through neurogenic tremors. If we can do this, the stress won't linger or manifest itself in a chronic way. Unfortunately, because our world is *so* stressful and *so* sedentary, we don't shift the stress quickly enough and it festers within us. Over the years, and if left unresolved, this festering emotional stress will cause a cascade of muscular tension. And, as we know, muscular tension creates imbalanced joints, which lead to muscular pain caused by imbalanced gravitational overload. As well as muscular pain, festering emotional stress and trauma can cause an alarming array of other physical and mental health conditions* Movement helps to process

* Wonderfully explored in books such as *The Body Keeps the Score* by Bessel van der Kolk and *When the Body Says No* by Gabor Maté.

and shift this stress and trauma out of the body before it causes harm.

One of the most beautiful things about improving your posture through corrective exercises is that it helps to tackle your mental state in several ways. Learning how to breathe and sit quietly with yourself while your joints are in a more comfortable, balanced and open position can immediately lower your stress levels. Tapping into diaphragmatic breathing is a simple way to immediately adjust your physiology and calm yourself in the moment. Balancing your joints, which we will explore in chapter 15, helps the systems of your body flow more effectively. The more often we return to the practice of moving our body in a gentle, compassionate and functional way – to improve the position of our joints and the function of our muscles – the less our body will be feeding the stress cycle.

Regular movement is pivotal to a calm nervous system. I truly believe improving posture is a powerful gateway to not only reducing physical pain but also lowering stress levels.

TAKEAWAYS

1. The nervous system controls our muscles, but our muscles also control the nervous system.
2. The nervous system and the muscles operate via the spinal cord.
3. Spinal alignment is critical to messages being delivered efficiently throughout the body.
4. My hunch is that spinal misalignment causes neurological conditions and many other types of condition.
5. Imbalanced posture can cause stress, and stress can cause imbalanced posture.
6. We can use posture exercises to help us tackle both stress and imbalanced posture, to bring our body into a calmer state.

CHAPTER 12
POSTURE AND THE DIGESTIVE SYSTEM

My hunch: Your posture impacts your digestive system

"Having worked with Ellie to improve my posture over the years, I have learned to breathe better, strengthen and release the muscles around my pelvis/hips and open up my ribcage.

These three things have helped tremendously with my IBS issues. Thank you, Ellie!"

Caroline

When we eat, our food enters the digestive system via the mouth, travels down the oesophagus into the stomach and moves through the intestines (fig. 43) until the remaining waste matter is passed out through the rectum. The waste passing out of the body is technically part of the excretory system, but I am going to bring the two together in this chapter.

Cast your mind back to the chapter on respiration. In chapter 9, I mentioned how your respiratory system (breathing) is impacted by the compressed torso position that occurs while sitting passively in a chair for a long period of time. I believe your digestive system to be no different.

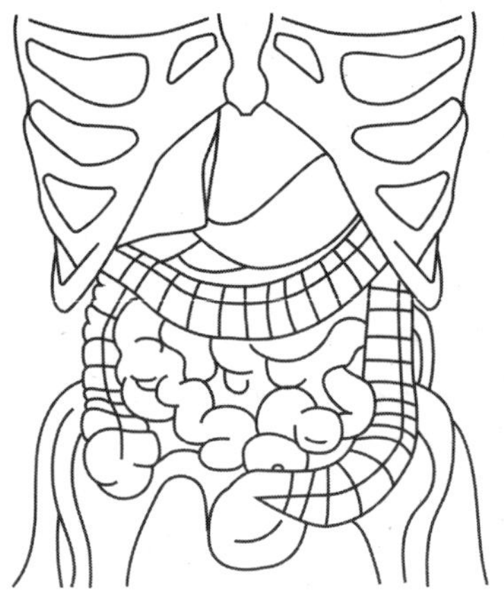

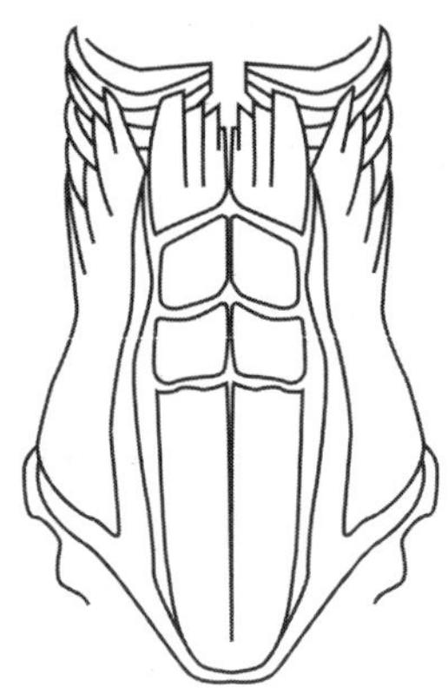

Figure 43a and b: The organs of digestion are housed within and around the superficial and deeper torso muscles. If these torso muscles are tense or imbalanced, it will exert an unnatural pressure on the organs of digestion housed within them.

As we become increasingly sedentary over time, our primary hip flexors – and other muscles close by, such as the abdominals and lower back muscles (fig. 43) – wind themselves up and become increasingly restricted and dysfunctional. These tense muscles eventually become so stuck and so dysfunctional that they cannot stretch themselves out again, even when we stand up. Consequently, the abdominal area remains in a perpetual state of compression and tension.

The hips and other torso muscles live under the same roof as the digestive system. So, the tension that is trapped in your hips is going to also pull on your organs of digestion. While many issues with digestion are caused by the type of food we eat and how stressed we are (yes, again!), I believe our digestive organs are being chronically compacted by our tense muscles. Our posture is impacting how comfortably our digestive system is sitting and, therefore, how well it is able to operate.

Over the years, I have lost count of the number of times I have given clients hip release posture exercises to free up their hip tension, and then heard feedback of gurgling bellies, farting and even a quick dash to the loo. Personally, I have no doubt that by releasing hip tension we can also immediately release gas and other substances trapped in the digestive system. Clients have anecdotally reported improvements in constipation and other digestive issues, such as IBS and gastric reflux, when they work on releasing the compression from their torso area and balancing their pelvis.

Undoubtedly, frequent movement helps us go to the loo. In the same way movement aids our immune and cardiovascular systems, by flushing lymph and blood around the body, movement helps with the efficient expulsion of waste matter. Those of us who spend time being active and upright will have much less of a fight against gravity when it comes to excretion. For those of who are sedentary, with a tucked pelvis, it is more likely that waste matter will linger for too long within the body.

Stop sucking in your belly
You need the freedom to breathe and move properly

As a young child, I did ballet until I was about eight years old. Attending ballet classes gave me a complex about my belly. I remember the ballet teacher shouting at me and repeatedly telling me to suck in my belly. Over the years, this created a subconscious movement pattern of belly clenching. It's only now that I am a movement teacher myself that I have realized this. To give my scary ballet teacher some grace, it wasn't only her instructions that gave me a fear of relaxing my belly. While I can't say I exercised a lot prior to finding my love for yoga, I did make some half-hearted efforts over the years to attend gym classes. During these various classes, from weightlifting to Pilates, I heard over and over again that we must "squeeze our core to protect our lower back". It's still a cue I routinely hear in my yoga and Pilates classes, but it's one with which I refuse to engage. Here's why.

As my knowledge of movement has grown, I have realized this cue is inherently damaging. Sucking in the belly does not protect the spine; it creates tension and stops us breathing functionally using our diaphragm. As you know, tension and dysfunction do not equal healthy movement patterns.

No part of our body is supposed to be held in a contracted state for much of the time. Muscles held in too much contraction become stiff and tense. Not good. Muscles are supposed to ebb and flow frequently through their full ranges of motion, and this creates mobility and mobility equals healthy movement patterns.

If you are habitually gripping your belly, for whatever reason, you are creating a situation in which you are less likely to have the toned belly or the strong spine you're after. A functionally toned belly is achieved through proper breathwork mechanics, full movement of the diaphragm, and frequent and varied movement of the ribcage, shoulders, pelvis and hips. That way, you are functionally engaging the muscles of your torso, without holding tension. If you are gripping your belly, you can't breathe properly or move your ribcage properly.

With regard to "squeezing your core to protect your lower back", habitual belly gripping creates compensation and overwork in the abdomen. In turn, this can encourage the lumbar, hip and pelvic muscles – which need to work in conjunction with the abdominal muscles to keep the spine aligned – to switch off and become dysfunctional. When you belly grip, it's highly likely you are also tucking your pelvis under posteriorly, flattening your lower back and creating hypertonicity (abnormally high muscle tone or tension) and brittleness in the pelvic floor. If the pelvis becomes stuck in the tucked under position, the muscles that are supposed to stabilize the pelvis and move the legs become dysfunctional. Thus, habitual belly gripping makes your spine more stiff and more vulnerable through the tension it breeds in the abdominal area and the instability it creates in the pelvis.

Personally, I have no idea where the "tuck your pelvis under to protect your lower back" or the "squeeze your core to protect your lower back" cues originated. Neither makes much sense in the context in which I hear them used. Yes, we want the ability to tuck our pelvis under when appropriate (such as when kicking a football up into the air), and yes, we want to be able to brace our core when appropriate (such as when lifting a heavy weight). But it's often not appropriate to cue these actions in yoga, Pilates and other exercise classes, and I spend a lot of time helping my clients unpick this learned movement pattern.

I teach my clients the benefits of releasing their belly (and, therefore, relaxing their brittle pelvic floor, which may be prone to leakages) and waking up all the muscles surrounding their belly area – which have switched off because the abdominals have taken over. It can be a real eye-opener to realize that the thing they were consciously doing to "help" themselves was actually one of the dysfunctional movement patterns causing more issues with pain and tension.

The reason I am focusing on belly gripping here is because the habit impacts the digestive system. Think about it, if we are sucking in the mass that is attached to our abdominal wall, where does that mass go? Inside our abdominal cavity. What is inside our abdominal cavity? Many of our vital organs. Just like the growth of a baby in the womb will displace some of our organs, frequently sucking in our belly also displaces some of our organs and puts too much pressure on them. The difference is that pregnancy is a non-permanent state of organ displacement, whereas belly gripping can become a life-long one. Over time, the pressure on our insides caused by belly gripping can create digestive issues, hernias and pelvic floor disorders. Belly gripping and intimidating ballet teachers have a lot to answer for!

Toilets are chairs
Our early ancestors didn't sit on a loo to poop

As mentioned previously, we need to reframe many of the things we consider normal. Only a few centuries ago, our ancestors did not have access to the modern technologies we use today. I've already discussed some of these, such as chairs, memory foam beds, baby bouncers, cars and padded shoes. I'm afraid to say that the humble seated toilet is another modern technology that strips movement from our body and impacts our digestive and excretive functions.

As a child I remember visiting countries like France, Spain and China on holiday, and being confused by all the squat toilets in the restaurants and service stations that we stopped at along the way. I used to be frightened of using them (I was convinced I'd make a mess) and did my best to avoid them at all costs, opting to wait until we got to the tourist-friendly hotel at our destination. For vast swathes of the world – although not the UK – the ubiquity of seated toilets is a relatively recent phenomenon. And there are places that still haven't introduced them widely.

Well, I was wrong to avoid squat toilets as a child, because squatting to toilet is far more beneficial for our health than sitting. Like it or not, human beings are designed to squat to defecate. This daily action, when performed in a squat, is not only the perfect natural mobility exercise to keep our ankles and hips mobile and strong, but it helps to clear the digestive tract more efficiently (fig. 44). As trapped faecal matter can lead to serious conditions like bowel cancer, the position we adopt is not to be taken lightly.

I am not suggesting you get rid of your toilet and dig a hole in the ground. However, it is useful to consider the benefits of squatting to toilet when looking at the bigger picture of how our modern environment is working so hard against what our body evolved to do. The more we can see the myriad ways our posture is being impacted by our environment – and not our genetics or age – the more it puts the power back in our hands to do something about it.

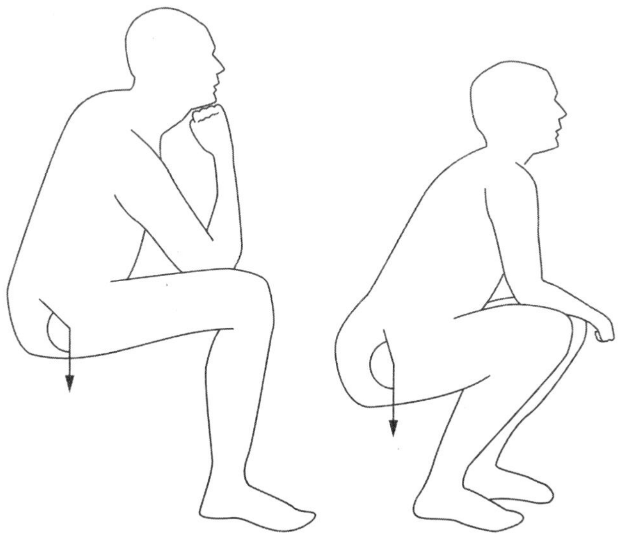

Figure 44: How a sitting position versus squatting position impacts how we squat.

If you want to create better excretion habits, you could try using a squatty potty, which is not as bad as you may think! It is a foot rest that elevates your feet so you are in a comfortable squatting position when you use the loo. Additionally, restoring the movement required (more ankle and hip strength and mobility) to be able to regularly practise the art of a "flat heels to the floor deep squat" will, among many other postural and movement benefits, help with your ability to expel waste matter more efficiently because the pelvis will be more aligned and engaged, which will help open the anal passage.

TAKEAWAYS

1. It makes sense to me that tension in the muscles within and around the torso and pelvis will pull on and compress the organs within the torso and pelvic region.
2. Releasing tension in the hips can cause gurgling, farting and sudden loo trips because muscular tension (and a lack of movement) traps gas and other waste materials inside the digestive tract for too long.
3. Being seated and sedentary prohibits the efficient movement of waste matter through the digestive system.
4. Belly gripping not only impacts your breathing and posture, but also compresses your internal organs.
5. Toilets are a modern technology. Squatting to toilet expels waste more efficiently.

CHAPTER 13
POSTURE AND THE REPRODUCTIVE SYSTEM

My hunch: Your posture impacts your reproductive system

My final hunch to explore in this book concerns the relationship between posture and the female reproductive system* I appreciate this is a sensitive topic, and they are many different factors that play a part in reproduction, pregnancy and birth. However, I felt I couldn't write a book about posture without sharing my thoughts on why I think our posture may be an important piece of the puzzle when we are preparing to reproduce.

I believe working on your posture before you try to conceive could be a game-changer in terms of how you experience the entire process, from conception to birth. Before I explain why I think this, I want to share a story from one of my long-term clients, who discovered posture in between her second and third pregnancies.

* I have helped male clients who have experienced numbness and a lack of function in their reproductive parts, but I have limited relevant experience working with males from which to draw conclusions about how postural imbalances impact their reproductive system. Because males are not carrying, growing and birthing the weight and size of a baby, I think postural imbalances probably impact their reproductive system less.

"As well as suffering less pelvic girdle pain during my third pregnancy and generally having an all-round more positive pregnancy experience, my third birth was amazing – I had the water birth I always wanted! When my contractions started in the morning, I did my full posture routine, meditation and breathwork. I felt like I knew how to work with my body to do what the muscles needed to do in each contraction and how to align my pelvis to make sure I wasn't holding any tension there. Trusting and knowing how to work with my body made the contractions less uncomfortable and more efficient.

My whole labour was much shorter and less hard work (than the previous two times) and I gave birth just a few hours later. I actually managed to 'breathe my baby out', which I thought was a lie until it happened to me! The midwives all said that the birth was pretty special and unusual to see.

I am convinced that my postural work made this possible for me, firstly due to better alignment of my pelvis but also due to a better connection with and understanding of my body. My change in mindset to trust my body allowed me to follow the natural process with confidence and understanding. The labour was a completely different experience to my other two, when labour was much longer and harder, and I had to be transferred to the ward for assistance.

I am now starting up some gentle posture exercises to help with recovery and an achy upper body from feeding round the clock – my body already feels stronger and in better alignment than previous recoveries though!"

Emma

The body needs to feel safe to reproduce
What is posture's role?

Reproduction is critical to the survival of the human race, but the reproductive system is not vital in terms of the day to day survival of an individual. Our body prioritizes other more essential functions, such as breathing, blood flow and the operation of other organs, before it can think about bearing a child. Many of us already know that the libido drops, hormones become disrupted, the menstrual cycle may stop and it can be harder to conceive when the body is under significant stress for a long time. The body is wise and, if already under a lot of stress, it recognizes that becoming pregnant and giving birth are going to add more stress to the mix. Therefore, the body prioritizes trying to restore homeostasis (a state of balance and stability) first.

The stress I describe above refers to general chronic life stressors, but I posit here that there is a relationship between the stress put on the body by imbalanced posture and how easily we are able to conceive, carry a child and give birth.

Before we conceive. As demonstrated in earlier chapters, the way in which dysfunctional imbalanced muscles stiffen around the hips and pelvis creates pelvic, hip and spinal postural imbalances. It is within this region that the female reproductive system is housed. So, if that housing is misaligned (because of a pelvic imbalance such as a hip hike), extremely tense (because of tight hip flexors that can't extend) and/or frequently compressed (because we spend a lot of time sitting down), it makes sense that the reproductive system is going to struggle to function optimally.

From client feedback over the years, I know that posture work can ease symptoms of intense, sometimes debilitating, stomach cramps that often accompany pre-menstrual syndrome. This may be because gentle, mindful, breathwork-focused posture exercises help to soothe the nervous system and put the body in a more relaxed state, or it may be because

I place heavy emphasis on restoring pelvic balance and freeing up tense hips. But there is a connection between posture work and easing of symptoms. It's not a coincidence. Personally, I feel a big difference when I have been slacking with my posture exercises: I am aware that my hips feel more restricted, and I experience more cramping in the run-up to/during my period.

If tension in the hips and pelvic area bears an undue pressure on the reproductive system that can exacerbate the intensity of menstrual cramps, my hunch is that there is a connection between this same postural pressure and other issues in the same system. If the reproductive system senses a great deal of unnatural imbalanced tension and pressure bearing down on it, combined with a nervous system on high alert due to the stresses of modern everyday life, is the body able to discern that this is not an optimal environment in which to conceive? I believe so.

Does the pregnancy itself cause the pain? I am convinced that the same common postural problems of pelvic imbalance and hip tension will create a painful pregnancy, with issues such as pelvic girdle pain and lower back pain. Most of the time, the postural issues exist prior to the pregnancy, but the extra load of the growing baby allows the mother to more intensely feel the symptoms of this postural imbalance. I appreciate that a hormone called relaxin and a protein called elastin are created during pregnancy, which helps to stretch out all the joints to create more space for the baby, and this will make the area more unstable. However, in the same way I don't believe increasing age causes pain, I don't believe pregnancy causes pelvic girdle pain: it's correlation not causation. If pregnancy caused pelvic girdle pain, everyone would experience it, and at the same stage of pregnancy. In my opinion, it is the combination of pelvic imbalance and added weight (from the growing baby) that causes pelvic girdle pain – not pregnancy itself.

An easier exit. Continuing in the same vein – I believe pelvic imbalance and tension around the hips puts a great deal of stress on the reproductive system, impacting its optimal function and efficiency – I believe the muscular function and position of the pelvic area will help to move the baby into an optimal position for birth and make labour more comfortable and efficient for both mother and baby. If the hips are mobile and free, the vaginal opening is going to widen for an easier exit. If the spine is mobile and the vertebrae are well aligned, the impact of pressure on the spinal column will be less painful. Control of the breath and diaphragm is also important for so many factors during labour: it helps with relaxing muscular tension as you experience contractions, optimal breathing to keep you and the baby calm, and pushing the baby out in the final moments of birth. Also, physiologically, giving birth is about working with the muscles in contractions and not fighting against what those muscles are trying to do. So, if you align your breathing, then you allow your diaphragm and pelvic floor to work together as intended.

There are no guarantees that posture work will give you what you want from conception through to birth, but I hope that my hunch makes sense to you in theory, and becomes yet another reason to consider working on your posture. There is nothing bad that can happen from getting your body more aligned – in less pain, stronger and more functional – but there is so much potential for unexpected positives to come from making some changes.

POSTURE EXERCISE

Releasing tight hips with the *Supine Groin Stretch*

Note: This exercise is not recommended if you are in the second trimester of pregnancy or beyond. If this is you, please revisit the posture test in chapter 1 (pages 12-14). That exercise will still stretch your hips but you won't be lying supine on your back.

One of my favourite posture exercises is Supine Groin Stretch. It is super relaxing and it is accessible to most of us. This exercise is a great way to reduce the hip flexor tension and pelvic imbalance that I have mentioned throughout this chapter. I suggest this exercise to clients who ask for advice on pre-menstrual syndrome stomach cramps (and also many other symptoms such as back pain, shoulder pain and knee pain).

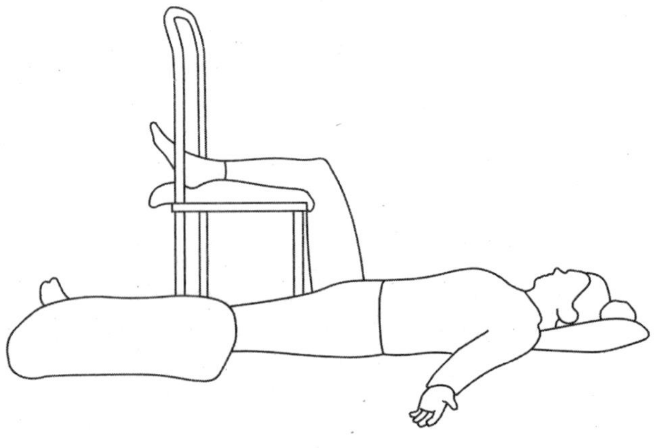

Figure 45: Supine Groin Stretch - You'll need your knee supported at a right angle over a chair and your outstretched leg supported by an object to stop it rolling out.

The reason I like this exercise so much is that I am yet to meet someone who, in my opinion, wouldn't benefit from relaxing their hip flexor muscles. It's not really possible to sit on a chair for most of the day for most of your life and not have tense hip flexor muscles. Therefore, this exercise can benefit most of us by relaxing our hips, balancing our pelvis, freeing our spine and repositioning our shoulders behind our body. Supine Groin Stretch can ease muscular tension and joint pain across all the joints in the body, because tension in the hip flexors has that much of a bearing on the rest of us. And because having tense hips is so influential, doing this exercise a few times a week can improve issues with digestion, breathing, circulation, constipation and pre-menstrual syndrome and so on.

1. Organize a set-up where you can lie on the floor and place one leg on something – a sofa, dining room chair or coffee table normally work well – and have a 90-degree angle at the hip and the knee (fig. 45). The bent leg needs to be able to relax without flopping inward or outward. Keep the kneecap in alignment with the hip joint, even when you're relaxed. Place cushions under your calf to help you achieve this.
2. Stretch the other leg out long. This leg needs to relax but not flop out to the side, so make sure you have something to prop against it. This could be a yoga bolster, some sturdy books or the edge of a low table.
3. Relax your lower ribcage and head into the floor and let your abdominal muscles go – no belly gripping. If you notice your lower ribcage is lifted off the floor or your chin is tilted upward to shorten the back of your neck, grab a pillow or two to help lower the ribcage and create more length down the back of the neck.
4. Place your arms away from your body, at about 45 degrees, palms facing up. All you need to do now is breathe through your nose, deeply into your diaphragm, and try and relax everything else. This exercise will not work if you are holding anything in your hands, so no phone and no reading. Meditating or listening to a podcast or music is perfect.
5. Spend at least 15 minutes in this position with one leg raised before swapping sides. Most of us will need a lot longer than 15 minutes on each side before our hips start to relax. You will know when this is happening because your lower back will naturally begin to touch

the floor without you gripping your belly or rolling your pelvis backward.

6. As with all posture exercises, your experience of Supine Groin Stretch will greatly evolve over time. The first time you do the exercise will hopefully yield an immediate sense of less pain and greater freedom, but the true benefits will only be felt with consistent practice. If you don't feel anything while doing this exercise, you probably don't have perfect hips! It's more likely that your hips are so tight that they need even more time on each side to start to relax.

Don't be alarmed if you hear your belly gurgling, experience some shaking or cramping muscles, need to rush to the loo, feel warmth and tingling spreading all over your body or experience strange new sensations going on during or after the exercise. All these may be positive and encouraging signs that your body is changing its alignment and that Supine Groin Stretch is a good exercise for you to practise.

If your symptoms of pain or tension are aggravated, try doing the exercise a little differently. You could:

- Use more or fewer pillows under your head
- Try two rolled-up towels under your neck and lower back, instead of a pillow under your head
- Start with the other leg first

If the exercise still doesn't feel good, leave it alone. It's not the one for you, and your body is telling you that you need to work on other bits of your posture first, before you try to relax your hips like this. In part 4, I'll help you to better understand these types of signals from your body.

Does your pelvic tilt impact the length of your pregnancy?

Is your pelvis telling your body when to go into labour?

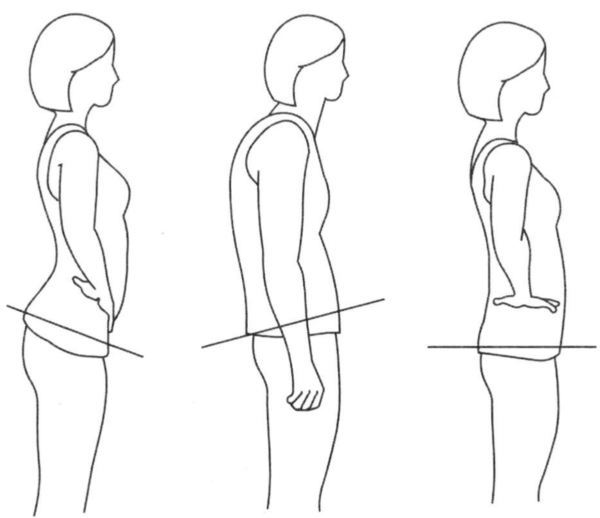

Figure 46: Anterior pelvic tilt, posterior pelvic tilt and neutral pelvic tilt.

In an ideal world, while standing, our pelvis would hold itself in what is considered a neutral pelvic position (fig. 46). A neutral pelvis means the top of the front of the pelvis and the back of the pelvis are more or less level (the black line) when viewed from the side. An anterior pelvic tilt occurs when the hip flexors in the front of the leg lock on and overpower the hip extensor muscles, such as the glutes, hamstrings and calves. A posterior pelvic tilt occurs when neither the hip flexors nor the hip extensors have enough strength to hold the pelvis in a stable position, and it tucks under. We want our pelvis to be able to flow between these two different pelvic positions, but, in a standing posture, your pelvis should be neither too tucked under nor too rolled forward: neutral.

In pregnancy, the pelvis naturally tilts forward into a more anterior pelvic tilt. This is due to the weight of the growing baby and it occurs to ready both the body and the baby for the process of giving birth, as the anterior pelvic tilt creates more space for exit through the vagina. Fascinatingly, for this exact purpose, the female body has three reinforced lumbar vertebrae, whereas the male body only has two. The extra reinforced vertebra helps to keep the spine happy during pregnancy.

Now, this is pure conjecture – I have not found scientifically supported data to support this theory put forward by Pete Egoscue – but I agree with Egoscue and believe having a "stuck" anterior pelvic tilt prior to pregnancy will impact not only the comfort and ease of pregnancy, labour and birth, but also whether the baby is carried to term. If an anterior pelvic tilt is a signal to the body that the baby is almost ready to be born, does it not make sense that a pre-pregnancy anterior pelvic tilt will become more anterior during pregnancy than nature intended? And could becoming too anterior too early in a pregnancy be a cause of some premature births?

Conversely, I believe the opposite could also impact whether a baby is overdue. If the body is already "stuck" in a posterior pelvic tilt before the pregnancy, I think the pelvis is more likely to struggle with the journey into an anterior position when the time is right. If the body does not receive the anterior pelvic tilt signal that the baby is almost ready to be born – the pelvis is staying tucked, which compresses the vaginal passage – I think it makes sense that the birth is more likely to be delayed in some way. Also, perhaps a body stuck in too much of a posterior pelvic tilt prior to birth is going to struggle, more generally, with giving birth naturally because there is less space available in the pelvic region?

I can't answer definitively on these theories and I can't find much by way of anyone else thinking this, but these hunches make sense to me and perhaps warrant further exploration.

I DON'T TEACH KEGELS (PELVIC FLOOR EXERCISES)

Kegels (or pelvic floor exercises) involve the contractions of muscles within the genital area.

I get asked a lot about pelvic floor exercises, but personally I don't teach them. My reasoning is I think pelvic floor exercises are overprescribed because we are focusing on a symptomatic area (symptom chasing), without considering the movement of the body more holistically. As with many musculoskeletal symptoms, the assumption is often that if there is a pelvic floor issue, there is a pelvic floor "weakness" that needs to be strengthened.

Often the pelvic floor leaks because it is brittle. What does "brittle" mean? Overworking and tense; compensating and exhausted. In many cases, I believe pelvic floor exercises exacerbate pelvic floor issues by making the pelvic floor more brittle and, therefore, more to prone to leakages. If there is no "give" in a structure, it is more likely to snap. Buildings in earthquake zones have a degree of wobble and movement built into them, so they don't collapse.

The pelvic floor can become brittle because it is working too hard on behalf of the diaphragm, hips, feet and glutes, which have become dysfunctional. For example, when the glutes are dysfunctional, we may instead tense our pelvic floor to compensate for the glute weakness. In a class, if I give the cue "squeeze your glutes, but not your pelvic floor", at least a few people (often those with pelvic floor leakage problems) will realize their pelvic floor is responding, not their glutes. But the pelvic floor is not designed to do the work of the glutes, and will become exhausted and dysfunctional too if this movement pattern continues. When a client has a pelvic floor issue, I find the best results come from teaching them to relax their pelvic floor (so it can become spongy and malleable again), breathe correctly using the diaphragm (which helps to stabilize the abdominal vacuum in which the pelvic floor resides), move their ribcage more functionally (which also helps to stabilize the abdominal vacuum), balance their hips and pelvis (to create support for the abdominal vacuum) and strengthen the muscles around their feet, hips and pelvis. There may well be some merit in some of us performing pelvic floor exercises (if the cause of the pelvic floor leakages is indeed weakness rather than overwork), but these exercises are already, in my opinion, so overprescribed and overrated that I prefer to offer alternative options to restore the integrity and function of the abdominal vacuum.*

* *Diastasis Recti* by Katy Bowman is a great book for understanding how pelvic floor issues are often a symptom of a whole body movement problem.

TAKEAWAYS

1. A body under stress will find is harder to conceive, because a stressed body will save its energy for more life-saving physiological functions.
2. Stress comes in different forms. I believe that postural imbalance is a type of stress that sends a "I don't feel safe" message to the body.
3. Tension through the hips is one of the most common postural dysfunctions I encounter. The hip flexors span the area where the reproductive system is housed. Surely tension here must impact the reproductive organs within?
4. I believe tension in the hips and imbalance around the pelvis make pregnancy more uncomfortable and a vaginal birth more complicated and painful.

5. A pregnant body naturally assumes a more anterior pelvic tilt in the later stages of pregnancy to facilitate birth.
6. If a pelvis (prior to pregnancy) is already anterior, does it increase the chances of an early arrival?
7. If a pelvis (prior to pregnancy) is already posterior, does this make it harder for the baby to come out and does it increase the chances of complications and a late arrival?
8 In my opinion, pelvic floor exercises are overprescribed and focus on the idea that the pelvic floor needs to be strengthened. The pelvic floor may actually be overworking and may need relaxing. You will be able to relax the pelvic floor by strengthening other parts of the body.

Conclusion

By this point in the book, I hope I have at least piqued your interest. I also hope you have a better understanding of what posture is and you appreciate the far-reaching impact your biomechanics may be having on unexpected aspects of your health and wellbeing. I assume you are ready and raring to go! I am an eternal optimist, and I do not intend to blame, scare or worry you at any point. My goals for you are ones of education and open-mindedness around reframing common narratives.

Trust in the healing power of your body and have faith that things can get a lot better than they are right now. Even if you feel pretty good at the moment, you will never regret future-proofing your body as soon as you can.

Brace yourself: the final section of the book is the hardest and most meaningful. Theory and education are all well and good, but theory means nothing if we do not try to change the habits that have led to our current situation. Part 4 offers you practical tips and posture exercises that will help you clarify which movement dysfunctions are causing your pain. While I would love you to feel changes almost immediately, these exercises are not a quick-fix solution. Nothing that works truly is.

This book is a mere springboard and introduction to posture. My exercises are intended to become a new lifestyle practice, something you do with the same regularity as brushing your teeth, drinking water or eating food. The hard part is not reading the book, but finding a way for the teachings of the book to seep into your everyday life. So, now is the time for commitment, self-compassion and the beginning of a life-long habit that will serve you today, next month and for the next 50 years.

PART FOUR
THE SOLUTION

CHAPTER 14

THE POSTURE TEN COMMANDMENTS

I deliberated long and hard about how much practical posture content to include in this book. It would have been easy to fill the pages with exercise walkthroughs, but it is difficult to capture the detail and nuance of my posture exercises through written word and diagrams alone. When teaching posture exercises, I always give elaborate amounts of verbal cueing (you've not experienced anything like it!), explaining the muscles you should and shouldn't be feeling, and I like to demonstrate the exercises myself, too. This is why I love using online video content to teach; it gives me the scope to do things properly.

Instead, in this book, I think it is more valuable for me to share my special posture diagnostic toolkit, my Function Tests (pages 201–217). These will enable you to further develop your understanding of the Posture Paradigm Shift (pages 57–63) – not symptom chasing but finding the root causes of your pain. Hopefully, by the end of part 4, you'll have identified which movement dysfunctions in your body are causing your symptoms of pain. You'll soon learn that dysfunction and pain are often in drastically different parts of the body (for example, a stiff dysfunctional foot can cause lockjaw). Armed with this new information, you'll then be able to better tackle your particular dysfunctions via my videos, in which I explain the posture exercises in the level of detail needed to succeed. Once you have finished the final section of the book, I will direct you toward the hundreds of free videos I have on my YouTube channel and to my website (page 231), so you can see how I can help you further.

Postural ground rules

Since I'm not there in-person to remind you, I need to hammer these ground rules home before you begin.

You need to take the following ground rules seriously. They are here to keep you safe and injury-free, and some of them are pivotal when it comes to understanding the Posture Paradigm Shift. It's amazing how many of us find these simple rules difficult, mainly because we live in a world where we have had the (unhelpful) phrase "No pain, no gain" shoved down our throats too many times. If you utter or even think these words to yourself, please give yourself a slap on the wrist from me. When it comes to reducing pain, we don't want to actively create pain by choice. That's obvious, right? From my experience, seemingly not!

1. Pain is to be respected

Pain is a message from your body asking you to listen to its wisdom. If you ignore this message and push through your pain, you will make your pain worse. If you continue to do exercises that aggravate your "normal" symptoms of pain (we will come to these after you've read these Ten Commandment) even a tiny bit, you are not respecting your body. You must immediately stop doing anything avoidable that makes you feel even marginally more tense or in pain in a "normal" way. Your body knows best; listen to it.

2. Hard work is intense but not painful

When you wake up dormant dysfunctional muscles, strange things can happen. You may wobble, cramp or burn, feel hot in the face or experience other unfamiliar sensations. These sensations are all good, provided you are not aggravating your normal symptoms of pain, because they are signs you are changing your posture. Change can be intense and it is rarely comfortable, but the hard work involved should feel different from your normal pain.

3. Maintain a calm breath, always

If you cannot maintain a calm, deep, nasal, diaphragmatic breath while exercising, you are pushing your body too hard. If you notice you are mouth breathing, holding your breath, clamping down on your jaw or raising your shoulders up around your ears, you're compensating using your breath. This means you are using unnecessary, forceful and compensatory tension in your upper body, neck and jaw – rather than functional muscles – to drive the movement. If you exercise like this, not only do you reinforce compensation (cheating) in your body (which will make you more tense), but you also send signals to your nervous system that you are not safe with what you're doing. Want to reduce your pain? Observe your breath when you exercise and keep it at a calm level. That way you will stop sending messages to your nervous system that it needs to be on high alert. Watching your pain levels and your breath are top priorities.

4. Don't force anything

When you exercise, if you are forcing, yanking, cranking or pushing, you'll end up hurting yourself. If your body likes what you're doing, you won't need to force it.

5. Do not symptom chase; find the root cause

If you symptom chase (focus on the part of your body that hurts), you'll end up frustrated and, most likely, in more pain. For example, if you have a painful lower back, do not do exercises or stretches that focus on the lower back (you can insert any part of your body here to make it relevant to you). This is symptom chasing. Leave the painful areas alone and concentrate on waking up the bits you don't often feel (in terms of pain or tension). When you wake up the sleepy bits, the overworking painful compensating parts will finally breathe a sigh of relief. Remember, don't poke the bear and all that. The Function Tests in chapter 15 will help you apply this concept.

6. Short-term changes happen quickly when you're on the right track

There's a myth that alleviating pain takes time. This belief is partially incorrect because short-term changes can and will happen immediately when you're doing the right exercise for your body. The myth is perpetuated because when we are trying to reduce pain, most of the time we are barking up the wrong tree (as per Commandment 5). For most pain, if you are doing an exercise that correctly tackles the root cause of your pain, you will immediately reduce your symptoms short term. When this happens, it's a sign you're on the right track. If your pain stays the same or gets worse, you're not doing the best exercise for your particular circumstance.

7. But ... long-term changes take time

Rewiring and strengthening all the muscles in your body long term – so the pain stays at bay for longer and longer periods of time – takes patience, perseverance and time. Posture work is a marathon, not a sprint. You will need to manage your expectations, especially if you have had pain or tension for more than a few months. Long-term changes will take time to take hold within your body.

8. Less is (generally) more

Some of my exercises may not seem to be doing anything. All my exercises do *something*, but sometimes they are working subtly. If your body is riddled with pain and your posture is heavily imbalanced, all you may be able to manage (without aggravating pain) are very passive exercises. In our hectic world, some of the most powerful exercises are the ones in which we are "just" lying down letting gravity, our breath and time work their magic.

9. Don't compare yourself

I think one of the reasons many of us break Commandments 1 and 4 is because we are either comparing ourselves to where we used to be or comparing ourselves to someone else. Your body is at where it is at. You can either accept this fact and work with it, or refuse to accept it and continue to fight against your body's wisdom. One of these routes will lead you to more pain; the other will free you from pain.

10. You are not alone

The emotional strain that comes with pain, combined with a medical system that may send you on a wild goose chase and fail to improve your symptoms, can make you feel alone. I totally understand this. However, you are not alone, and there are plenty of people out there who feel the same as you. There are lots of people who have had pain that is the same as yours, and they have got better from it – or at least dramatically reduced it. Find a community that can support you, do your posture exercises with a friend or family member and stay hopeful. There is always hope.

CHAPTER 15
FUNCTION TESTS

The posture detective's self-diagnostic toolkit

Now we have got the all-important ground rules out of the way, you are ready to become a fully fledged posture detective. I will teach you how to use certain "tools" to detect the root causes of your pain, which will put you on the right track in terms of seeking out the most suitable posture exercises for your body. I call these tools "Function Tests".

The term "Function Tests" is just a fancy way of saying "exercises that teach you something about your muscular function". Here, I am going to share five of my favourite Function Tests. Typically, I find that one or more of these will give some clarity and direction to most posture detectives. If the Function Tests don't work for you, don't worry, I have some more tricks up my sleeve in the final section of part 4.

Stage one: Taking stock

To be able to track any changes that may occur in your body, you will first need to take stock of your starting point, and observe and make a note of the levels and areas of your normal symptoms of pain and tension while standing still.

Please take off your shoes and socks and come to a standing position. Shake out your arms and legs, march up and down, and then find stillness in your natural standing posture. By its nature, your natural standing posture does not involve any forced, stiff, self-conscious posing, so please remember to drop any notion of what you think "good" posture is. You are not to hold your breath, pull your shoulders back, widen your palms, adjust your collapsed feet or squeeze your belly or glutes; just relax and let your body be.

When you have established your natural standing posture, close your eyes, relax your breathing and begin to sense into your body. I want you to ask yourself several questions, and then afterwards write your answers down on a piece of paper. Your answers will help you to build your case file (understanding the root causes of your pain and tension) and gather evidence (determining which new muscular activations change the location and severity of your pain and tension) to help you find the culprit (the stiff weak dysfunctional parts of you that are causing the pain and tension). Be honest. You need to give yourself a subjective score out of ten.

ASSESSMENT

1. **Am I in pain? Where is the pain and how bad is it?**
   Example answer: I have right knee pain at 2/10 and neck pain at 4/10.
2. **Do I feel tension? Where is the tension and how bad is it?**
   Example answer: I have lower back tension at 5/10 and an awareness of my right quad gripping at 1/10.
3. **Do I have more weight in one leg than the other?**
   Example answer: I have slightly more weight in my right leg than my left leg.
4. **How are my feet interacting with the ground and do I feel stable?**
   Example answer: My feet feel collapsed in the arches. I have more weight through the front of my right foot, and I am swaying forward and backward.

5. **Can I get a sense of where my arms and shoulders are?** Example answer: I feel like my shoulders and arms are rounded forward, my right side more so than my left side.

Once you have established your starting point, you will be able to assess which of the Function Tests make the biggest impact on your posture.

Note: Some of you may report you do not detect any pain, tension or imbalance. I am yet to meet anyone where this is truly the case. It may be that you are not (yet) able to tune into this type of assessment, or that you have become so used to underlying pain, tension or imbalance that you no longer register the sensations. If you really don't feel anything, I'd still like you to do the Function Tests. Hopefully, when you reassess yourself at the end, you'll sense changes and realize you did have some imbalances when you started.

Stage two: Function Tests

Before you begin, please bear in mind there are three possible outcomes for each Function Test.

Outcome 1: The Function Test makes your pain/tension feel better.
Outcome 2: The Function Test makes your pain/tension feel worse.
Outcome 3: The Function Test makes no impact on your pain/tension.

You are looking for Outcome 1. If any of the Function Tests gives you an Outcome 1, it means you have identified the part of your body you need to address first to reduce your pain/tension. (See each Function Test below for further explanation.)

As previously mentioned, improvements can be very subtle, but they are still improvements. For some of us, a Function Test may immediately take away all symptoms of pain, and so seem quite miraculous. For others, there may still be some pain after doing the test, but it has reduced. This is still a positive sign. You may notice pain lessens in one part of your body, but stays the same in another. This is also a positive sign, and this outcome tells you that the remaining pain is probably caused by a different part of the body being dysfunctional. One of the other Function Tests may reveal where that problem lies.

If none of the Function Tests give you an Outcome 1, don't give up hope. I have chosen just five tests (of hundreds) to include in this book, and they do not cover all ranges of movement. Hopefully, the three posture exercises in chapter 16 will offer some insight and relief instead. If not, you've got some further posture detection work to do to discover which range of movement helps you the most. I suggest heading to my YouTube Channel and working your way through more of my instructional videos!

NOTE:

If any of the Function Tests (or previous posture tests in the book) make you feel good and reduce your pain/tension, please use them as posture exercises - to do as often as you like throughout your day.

Function Test 1: Standing pigeon-toed

Tests to see how changing your foot position/function changes your pain/tension.

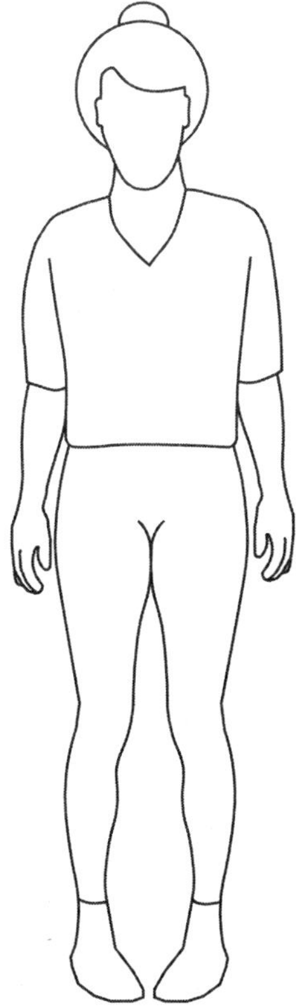

Figure 47: The Standing Pigeon-Toed test can be done at or away from a wall.

Stand in the middle of a room or against a wall. Standing against a wall will help you to reduce rotation through your pelvis, because you will get feedback from the wall if one butt cheek is further forward than the other.

For this test, all you need to do is turn your feet into a pigeon-toed position. Make sure you are not turning so pigeon-toed that you feel discomfort in the knees. Relax your toes, ensuring they are spread wide and flat. Pin into your big toe joints, rolling the arches of your feet down into the floor. Try and pin down equally between both feet.

Keep a little softness in your knees and focus on how your foot and ankle areas are starting to switch on. You may notice you tend to lock your knees back into hyperextension, which is one of the ways your body may try to avoid (compensate) the new foot function we are trying to create here.

Keep your calves, heels and bottom against the wall. Just like in the Standing at Wall posture test in chapter 1 (pages 12–14), don't thrust your shoulders, arms and head backward. Allow them to slump. Do your best to relax your upper body and your belly. Maintain calm, deep, nasal, diaphragmatic breathing. Try and stay here for up to five minutes, but take a break if it gets too intense.

If you get any aggravation of a normal symptom of pain/ tension, stop the test. If you feel your feet and lower legs working hard, cramping, going bright red or getting veiny, or any shakiness through the legs, these are all great signs your posture is changing.

At the end of the exercise, reassess your natural standing posture and ask yourself the same five assessment questions as before. Notice if anything has changed.

If you have an Outcome 1 somewhere in your body (the Function Test makes my pain/tension feel better), you now know that you should focus on improving the function of your feet if you want to reduce pain/tension in the part of your body that feels better.

Posture exercise prescription: Go to the end of the section and find the Wall Frog instructions (pages 221–222). See how ten minutes in Wall Frog makes you feel. Wall Frog creates change by altering the function and position of the feet and ankles. It is a logical next step if you found Standing Pigeon-Toed (or Standing at Wall) beneficial.

Function Test 2: Hands behind head
Tests to see how changing your thoracic (mid-back) and shoulder position changes your pain/tension.

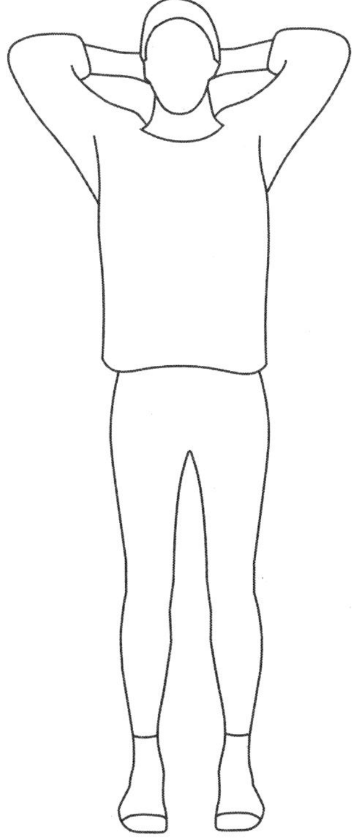

Figure 48: Make sure your feet stay parallel for the Hands Behind Head test.

Set your feet up as though you are standing on narrow train tracks, making sure you are not measuring your parallel foot alignment from the position of your big toe. The centre of each foot needs to face forward, not outward.

Interlink your hands and put them behind your head at the base of your skull, keeping the back of your neck long. Check you are not putting your hands on your neck. Keep your wrists in line with your elbows, not below.

Make sure you're happy that you're not aggravating any existing pain/tension in this position (if so, stop). Engage the muscles between and under your shoulder blades by pulling them together and down away from your ears. As you engage these muscles, your breastbone should not lift toward the ceiling. If it does, you're compensating with your spine rather than functionally moving your shoulders. Try again. Also make sure you don't poke your head forward; you don't want your neck to compensate for your dysfunctional shoulders.

Relax your belly and jaw. Maintain a calm, deep, nasal, diaphragmatic breath throughout. Hold this position for up to five minutes, stopping when necessary and trying to keep both shoulders equally engaged.

If you get any aggravation of a normal symptom of pain/tension, stop the test. If you feel your arms, shoulders, upper back or mid-back burning and working hard, these are all great signs your posture is changing.

Note: Pins and needles are common during this Function Test. This outcome tells you that your arms cannot rotate functionally within the shoulder joints. Stop the exercise if you get pins and needles.

At the end of the exercise, reassess your natural standing posture and ask yourself the same questions as before. Some things may be the same, but others may have changed.

If you have an Outcome 1 somewhere in your body, you now know that you should focus on improving the function of your shoulders and thoracic area if you want to reduce pain/tension in the part of your body that feels better.

Posture exercise prescription: Go to the end of the section and find the instructions for Static Back (pages 218–219) and Modified Floor Block (pages 220–221). See how ten minutes in either of these makes you feel. Static Back and Modified Floor Block create change by altering the function and position of the ribcage and shoulders. Either is a logical next step if you found Hands Behind Head beneficial.

Function Test 3: Standing on one leg

Tests to see how bearing more load through your less dominant leg changes your pain/tension.

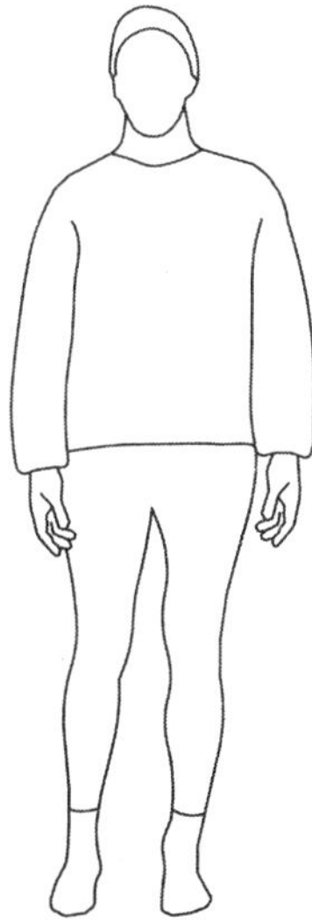

Figure 49: Stand with more weight on your less dominant leg.

WHICH IS MY LESS DOMINANT LEG?

Have a look back at your answers to the assessment questions. Did you report that you bear more weight through one leg than the other? Do you normally suffer symptoms of pain/tension in one leg but not the other? If so, you have an easy answer. Your less dominant leg is the one that bears less weight or is less symptomatic. Choose that leg for the next Function Test.

If you felt balanced when you did the assessment and you don't have one-sided leg symptoms, do the following test for two and a half minutes on each side and see which leg works harder when under load. The leg that is working harder is your less dominant leg.

For this exercise, shift your pelvis sideways so you are bearing more weight through your less dominant leg. Please note that shifting your pelvis sideways does not mean tipping your upper body sideways.

As in the Standing Pigeon-toed test, spread your toes wide and flat and keep them relaxed. Pin into your big toe joint and keep a softness at the knee joint to prevent any potential knee hyperextension (compensation).

Relax your belly and jaw. Maintain a calm, deep, nasal, diaphragmatic breath throughout. Hold this position for up to five minutes.

If you get any aggravation of a normal symptom of pain/tension, stop the test. If you feel your weight-bearing leg is burning and working hard, possibly all the way from toes to glutes, this is a great sign your posture is changing.

At the end of the exercise, reassess your natural standing posture and ask yourself the same questions as before. Some things may be the same, but others may have changed.

If you have an Outcome 1 somewhere in your body, you now know that you should focus on teaching your less dominant leg to bear more of your weight if you want to reduce pain/tension in the part of your body that feels better.

Posture exercise prescription: Go to the end of the section and find the instructions for Static Back (pages 218–219) or Wall Frog (pages 221–222). See how ten minutes in either of these makes you feel. Static Back and Wall Frog are both good for creating pelvic balance, which helps to realign the hips and so balance out weight distribution. Either is a logical next step if you found Standing on One Leg beneficial.

Function Test 4: Standing glute squeeze
Tests to see how more glute function changes your pain/tension.

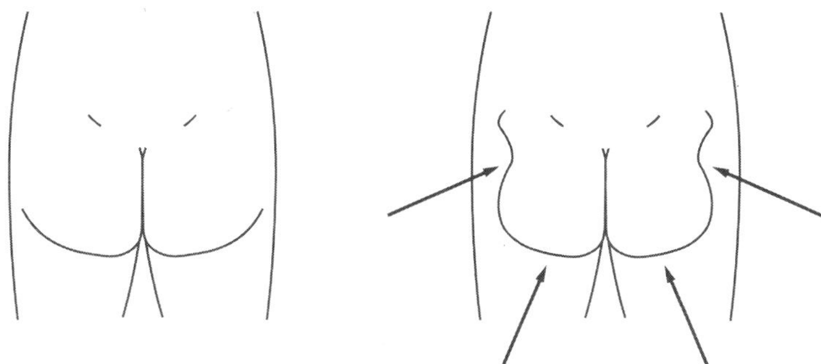

Figure 50: A glute squeeze is surface level and can be felt if you place your hands on your butt.

Assume the same parallel standing position as for Hands Behind Head and squeeze your glutes (butt muscles). Hold this position for up to five minutes.

Please note that your glutes are not your quads, your abdominals or your pelvic floor. As our glutes lose function – this happens when we sit on them too much – our quads, abdominals and/or pelvic floor often learn to compensate on their behalf. You will know you are squeezing your glutes because you'll be able to feel the muscles contract if you place your hands on your butt.

If you get any aggravation of a normal symptom of pain/ tension, stop the test. If you feel your glutes waking up and working hard, and possibly wobbles through your legs, this is a great sign your posture is changing.

At the end of the exercise, reassess your natural standing posture and ask yourself the same questions as before. Some things may be the same, but others may have changed.

If you have an Outcome 1 somewhere in your body, you now know that you should focus on waking up your glutes if you want to reduce pain/tension in the part of your body that feels better.

Posture exercise prescription: Go to the end of the section and find the instructions for Wall Frog (pages 221–222) See how ten minutes in Wall Frog makes you feel. Wall Frog creates change by putting the hips into external rotation and abduction (which are some of the roles of the glutes). Wall Frog is a logical next step if you found Standing Glute Squeeze beneficial.

Function Test 5: Standing chest opener

Tests to see how improving your hand function changes your pain/tension.

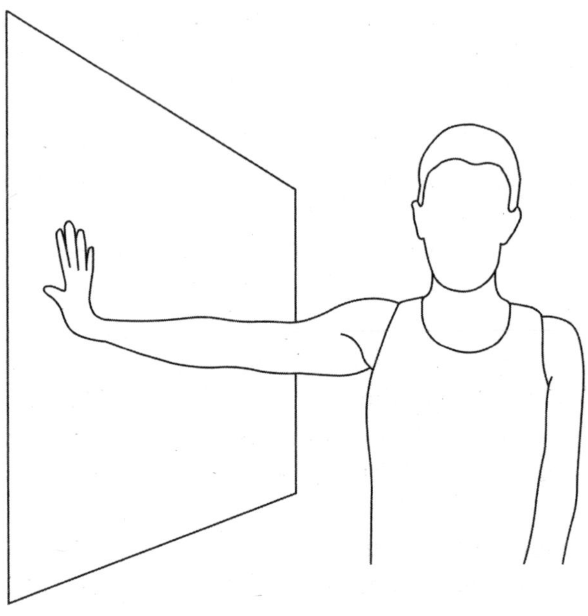

Figure 51: Chest Opener - Stand parallel to a wall, fingers outstretched and flat to the wall, and hold.

Stand sideways to a wall and make sure you can put your hand flat against the wall. Spread your fingers wide, so you can feel a stretch in the palm of your hand and between your fingers. Your hand should be at about shoulder height, but if you have wrist pain when you do this, place your hand a bit higher instead. If this still feels painful, stop the exercise.

Stand with the same parallel foot alignment as before, spreading your weight evenly through the length of both feet. Make sure you keep your weight evenly distributed throughout the exercise, because you may notice you start to avoid the foot closest to the wall once the hand starts to stretch. This is the body trying to compensate away from the tension in the hand.

Keep a soft bend in your elbow and focus on the hand stretching. Make sure you don't hyperextend your elbow to compensate for hand dysfunction. Once you can feel your hand stretching – the sensation may radiate up into the forearm – pull your shoulder blade back and down away from your ear, without thrusting the breastbone upward. If the hand and arm are tense, you may notice your shoulder shoot up around your ear. If your shoulder is dysfunctional, the ribcage may lift as compensation for the shoulder being asked to pull down. Keep your ribcage parallel to the wall to open up the front of the chest, and make sure the ribcage is not twisting toward the wall.

Hold this position for up to five minutes before swapping sides. You will probably find it particularly difficult to maintain the calm, deep, nasal, diaphragmatic breathing. I need you to find your edge and maintain a level of hand stretch where the breath can remain calm. This will likely come from bending the elbow a little more.

Note: Pins and needles are common during this Function Test. This outcome tells you that your arms cannot rotate functionally within the shoulder joints. Stop the exercise if you experience pins and needles.

If you get any aggravation of a normal symptom of pain/tension, stop the test. If you feel burning and intense stretching in your hands, forearms, upper arms and shoulders, and possibly wobbles through your arms and torso, this is a great sign your posture is changing.

At the end of the exercise, reassess your natural standing posture and ask yourself the same questions as before. Some things may be the same, but others may have changed.

If you have an Outcome 1 somewhere in your body, you now know that you should focus on your tense hands and wrists if you want to reduce pain/tension in the part of your body that feels better.

Posture exercise prescription: Go to the end of the section and remind yourself of the instructions for Modified Floor Block (pages 220–221). See how ten minutes in Modified Floor Block makes you feel. Modified Floor Block creates change by opening up the front of the chest and stretching out tight arms. This posture exercise is a logical next step for someone who found Standing Chest Opener beneficial. But also, keep repeating this Function Test as an exercise. Standing Chest Opener is a great one to do at work to offset typing and phone "claw hands".

Assessing your outcomes

For some of you, this last task may seem a little unnecessary. But as a posture therapist, I have learnt that Function Test theory needs to be repeated time and time again, and it still sometimes doesn't sink in. The theory is not complicated, but it generally goes against a lifetime of symptom chasing, so it can be difficult to absorb and understand.

To help you see things more clearly, and in terms of your own body, here is a "fill in the blanks" crib sheet to use for all the Function Tests. Copy it out, and then fill it in – one for each Function Test. Stick up your completed crib sheets somewhere visible so you don't forget what you learned.

Where I have left blanks, insert the pain/tension you noted during your original Assessment. Where it is bold in the text, insert the relevant outcomes and body parts according to the Function Test you're evaluating. I have written the crib sheet in the singular in terms of pain/tension. Please use plural pains/tensions if this is relevant to your body.

FUNCTION TEST CRIB SHEET

Grab some paper and write this down.

I have pain or tension in my _______________. This pain/tension is there because that part of my body is overloading or overworking on behalf of something else and it's tired and worn out. This area of my body is not the problem; it is a victim of compensation. I must leave this part of my body alone to rest (to the best of my ability), so I don't make it overwork more than needed.

If I have pain/tension in my _______________ then repeatedly trying to strengthen or stretch this area of my body will make it overwork and feel worse. I am symptom chasing.

When I did **Function Test 1 (which tests for foot dysfunction)**, my pain/tension improved/got worse/stayed the same. If my pain/tension improved, this tells me that **my dysfunctional feet** cause the compensatory pain/tension in my ____________. To reduce the compensatory pain/tension in my _____________, I need to work on improving **the function of my feet.**

TAKEAWAYS

For some of you, the Function Tests (although maybe challenging) will have made you feel good more generally, and doing the exercises will have reduced your normal symptoms of pain/tension. If so, improving your posture should be quite simple. You need to take a whole body approach to improving your muscular function, and then everything will feel much better with time and a regular posture practice. As you work on a bit of everything, your body will slowly balance itself out and move more efficiently. The Function Tests and exercises in this book are a great place to start, but they are just the tip of the iceberg.

For others of you, whose bodies are typically more dysfunctional and/or have suffered for longer, I would not advise taking a whole body approach initially. Although everything in your body is probably dysfunctional to some extent, and eventually each area will need a lot of work, the order in which you approach things is crucial to improving your posture successfully. It's about finding the right knot in the string to tackle first (remember my ball of string analogy earlier?). For a tightly wound-up body, you can't start picking apart knots in the middle of the string. Posture progress doesn't work like that.

In some respects, it's easier if only one or two of the Function Tests improved your normal symptoms of pain because it's more obvious where to concentrate your attention. In this situation, the difficulty - in my experience - is the mindset, not the body. Some of us don't like to focus narrowly on one part of the body, especially if it's not the bit where we are experiencing pain/tension. I think this is largely down to anxiety that we are "not doing enough". Let me reassure you: if you show up for yourself in a compassionate way, nearly every day, over several months, practising exercises that make you feel even marginally better, you *are* doing enough - even if you aren't going through a varied or huge range of different posture exercises.

If this is you, remember numbers 6, 8 and 9 of The Posture Ten Commandments.

1. When you are on the right track, your pain will reduce quickly. Stay on that path, even if that track seems narrow to begin with.
2. Sometimes, all that is needed (or is possible) is consistency in your practice and compassion for yourself.
3. You can only ever meet your body where it is right now. Respect this, and don't compare yourself to where you were before or what you think you should be able to do.

If only one of the Function Test reduced your pain, stay in this lane. You'll be ready to branch out soon enough, but only if you learn to respect the order and speed at which your body needs to unravel. As you gently relax and release your joints and muscles in the right order (for you), you will notice your capabilities (how many posture exercises you can do without aggravating pain and tension) start to dramatically expand. Let the wisdom of pain be your guide and don't let the delusion of ego steer you off-track.

CHAPTER 16
YOUR STARTER POSTURE KIT

Three posture exercises you can do every day

Some of you may have looked through this book hoping to find a chapter titled "Fixing Knee Pain", for example, with exercises to follow. But the root causes of knee pain are not the same for all of you, so that format wouldn't work. There is no such thing as a universally helpful routine for any specific symptom, because an exercise that improves knee pain for some could make it worse for others. If you have knee pain due to a rounded upper body position (tipping the weight forward onto the front of the feet and overloading the knees), you need to practise upper body exercises. But if you have knee pain because your hip flexors are weak (losing stability at the pelvis and overloading the knees), you need hip strength exercises in your practice. You can see my predicament and why I decided to focus on showing you how to detect the root causes of your pain instead. With this information about your body, you can delve further into the world of posture by visiting body-part specific classes on my YouTube channel.

Before you go, here are my three favourite starter posture exercises. Technically, you now have my top six starter posture exercises, because I included my other three favourites in the earlier posture tests: Standing at Wall (pages 12–14), In-line Position (pages 125-128) and Supine Groin Stretch (pages 181–183).

The starter posture exercises each target the whole body (as do all posture exercises), but in different ways. By practising these exercises, you are doing a lot of good for the alignment of your musculoskeletal system, even though it may not seem like you are doing much. Expect some unfamiliar sensations (signs of postural change), but stop the exercise if it aggravates a normal symptom of pain (that is, the pain doesn't relax off after 30 seconds). Remember to maintain a calm, deep, nasal, diaphragmatic breath throughout.

Start by doing each exercise in isolation – not all in one go. This is so you can assess how you feel after each one and identify the variables. If you do all three exercises in a row and then notice your pain is aggravated, you won't be able to detect which exercise caused you grief. Do one exercise a day over a three-day period, and assess each one individually in terms of whether it suited your body.

You will see in the instructions below that you can potentially hold each of these exercises for 30 minutes. Please be aware that you may need to work toward this, and you may want to start off holding them for just a few minutes. Despite how simple the exercises look, they will dramatically remodel your posture. If you create too much change too quickly, the sensations you experience afterwards may be so intense you will be nervous to repeat the exercises. Slowly increase the amount of time you spend in each position, so you gently remodel your posture at a steady pace and build your confidence, too.

1. Static back

Purpose: Uses gravity for pelvic and ribcage balance, spinal length and alignment, shoulder and femur repositioning.

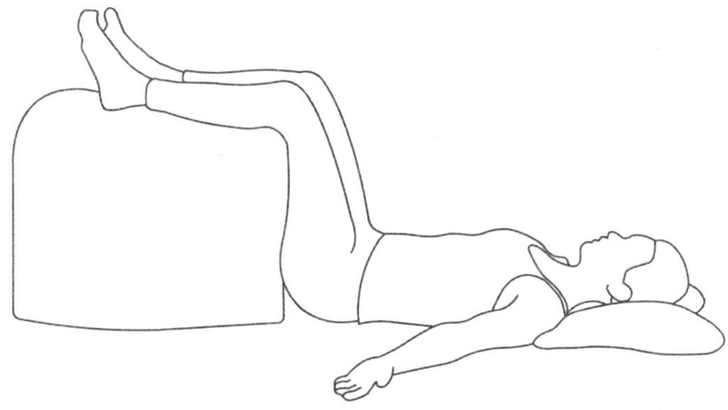

Figure 52: Static Back set up – calves need to be high enough that legs can fully relax but be supported at hip-width apart. Cushion to keep ribcage grounded.

A sofa works well for this exercise. Lie on the floor and shuffle up to the sofa so your bottom fits snug against it and your hips are at a 90-degree angle. Relax your legs, but don't allow them to flop in or out. If your legs flop out of alignment with your hip joints, put a cushion or two under your calves.

I recommend trying this exercise with two cushions under your head to start with, but stiff kyphotic (rounded) upper backs may need even more support. The purpose of the cushions is so you can keep the back of your neck long and your lower ribcage grounded. As you practise this exercise more often, and as your upper back lengthens, you will be able to reduce the number of cushions you need until eventually you can have your head directly on the floor. If you don't use cushions (when your body needs you to), you'll notice the bottom of your ribcage lifts off the ground, your shoulders are rounded forward off the ground and your head tilts backward, putting your neck into hyperextension. Your body will not be able release properly if you do not use cushions when you need to.

Turn your hands so your palms face upward and place your arms away from your body at about 45 degrees (not straight out at the shoulders). If this position feels good, stay here for up to 30 minutes.

2. Modified floor block

Purpose: Uses gravity to open the chest, reposition the shoulders, balance the pelvis and ribcage, lengthen the spine, plantarflex the feet and stretch the hips into extension.

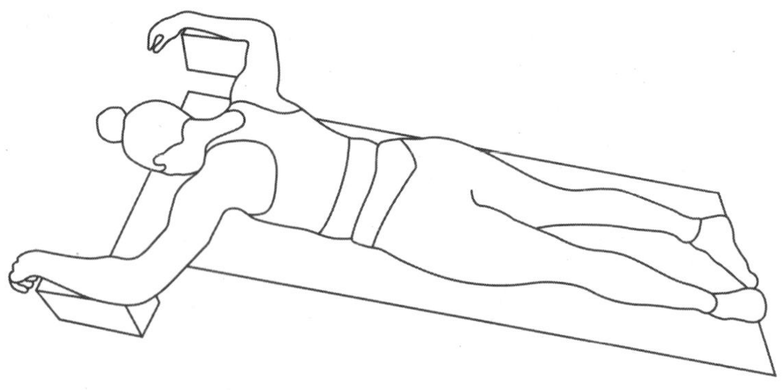

Figure 53: Modified Floor Block - Pigeon-toed feet, relaxed arms and legs, and deep breathing.

Use two identical yoga blocks for this exercise, or two shoe boxes or two piles of books. Set your blocks out at the side of your shoulders so there is a 90-degree angle at both your armpit and your elbow when you lay your forearm along the block in a cactus shape. Note that the yoga blocks are on the "medium" height, so the long thin edge of the block faces up to the ceiling. Bring your big toes together and allow the ankles to relax out to the side in a pigeon-toed position. Completely relax your whole body in this position; the only active part of you will be your deep breathing into the sides and back of your ribcage.

A common mistake in this exercise is putting your forehead on the ground, which will compress the nose and hyperextend the neck. You need to put the top of your head on the ground to allow your neck to lengthen and stretch. If this position feels good, stay here for up to 30 minutes.

3. Wall frog

Purpose: Uses supination and plantarflexion of the feet to open the hips into a more externally rotated and abducted position. Simultaneously, uses gravity to relax the pelvis, spine, ribcage and shoulders, much like Static Back.

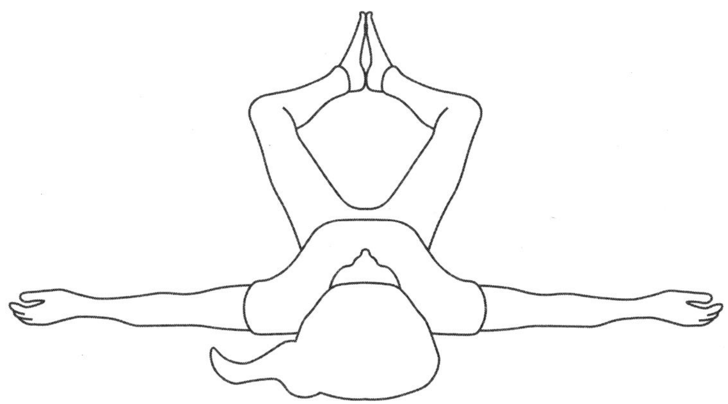

Figure 54: Wall Frog - The outside edges and balls of the feet stay connected as the feet push together constantly. The upper body relaxes and the pelvis stays grounded.

You need a wall for this one and probably a couple of cushions. As in Static Back, your lower back and ribcage need to remain grounded, so use cushions under your head if necessary. Your pelvis also needs to be fully grounded, so make sure you're not too close to the wall and lifting your tailbone off the floor. Bring the soles of your feet together, so there is a connection between the balls of the feet/big toe joints and the outer toes. If your ankles are stiff, you may struggle to touch the outer toes together, but do your best.

From here, gently and evenly push your feet together. As you push, make sure the big toes joints don't come apart, and try and keep the big toes themselves connected. You may notice you are pushing the tops of your feet away from you and into the wall. Try and feel like you are almost scooping the balls of the feet back toward you, while also pushing them together. Make sure one leg isn't dominant; we want both feet working evenly.

In this position, the feet are working quite hard and you may experience cramping and wobbling through your feet, calves, thighs and hips. This is good. Keep your upper body and breathing relaxed while the legs work hard. Hold this position for up to 30 minutes.

Sequencing

Once you have practised these exercises in isolation a couple of times and decided which ones work well for your posture, play around with sequencing them. For example, if you felt that waking up your feet in the Standing Pigeon-toed Function Test made the biggest difference to your posture, then start your sequence by waking up your feet in Wall Frog. Similarly, if putting your Hands Behind Head helped during the Function Tests, then starting your sequence with Modified Floor Block would probably work well for you. Once you've decided on a sequence, do each exercise for about ten minutes, creating a 20- to 30-minute posture sequence.

If only one of the starter posture exercises felt good for you, focus on that one. Keep practising the exercise and start holding it for longer and longer periods of time. Eventually, this foundational posture work will begin to open up further exercises for you.

If none of the three starter posture exercises felt good for you, well done for listening to your body's wisdom. Perhaps one of the earlier posture exercises in the book felt better? If so, focus on that one to begin with. If you are struggling to work out where to start, I suggest beginning in a standing posture, such as any of the five Function Tests, Standing at Wall or In-line Position.

CHAPTER 17
WHAT NEXT?

You are in charge and that's a good thing

I can't quite believe we are here, but it's time to wrap things up. I am going to finish the book with a final list of postural pointers, to help you improve your posture, reduce your tension and keep you away from devices of external support. But first, I want to speak about staying hopeful.

Some of you may feel a little despondent right now. A lot of the book has been about outlining how much our modern world works against our body. So how can we, or our children, ever feel good when everything in our everyday life is fighting against us? Our modern world and environment are what they are – for better and for worse – so we must learn to deal with them.

With this book, my intention is not to make you feel hopeless, but to inform and empower you to make better decisions to benefit you and your family. Believe me, there is *so much more* you can do to feel better than you do now, but you will need to make different choices – possibly difficult choices – to create change. A simple and common example of this would be to choose to walk up the stairs rather than ride up the escalator. An oldie but a goodie!

My final list of postural pointers offers you some more examples of decisions you can make, which will make a noticeable difference without taking up too much extra time.

Alongside making lifestyle changes, I'd like you to consider integrating a more conscious mobility and posture focused movement practice into your weekly schedule. (Ideally, this will become a daily schedule, but aim for three times a week at first.) It is relatively easy to change how much time we spend sitting down or to choose to wear a different type of shoe. However, for most of us, there will be a lot of remedial and repairing postural work that needs to happen routinely alongside our lifestyle changes.

Remember, the world has been acting against you in many ways from the moment you were born. If you're anything like me, your body will need a fair amount of posture work to restore its balance and improve its function to a more optimal level. Our environment no longer offers the natural stimuli we need to keep a human body healthy, so we must choose to carve out time to create this for ourselves. This is where a conscious movement practice comes in.

I have suggested some posture exercises to get you started, but there are hundreds more on my YouTube channel, and you can choose increasingly challenging exercises as your body becomes more functional. Strength and change come from challenge and different stimuli; you need to keep working hard and increasing the demand on your body so your progress doesn't plateau. So please don't be tempted into complacency once you have got rid of your pain. I realize you will be relieved you are feeling better, but you need to keep going; your pain will return and your body will regress if you do not make this type of work routine.

What do I want you to do?

First, I want you to recruit friends and family members to join your endeavour. We are social beings, and we are motivated by what our peers are up to. You will stick with your posture exercises for longer if others around you are also trying to create change. Can you create some accountability for yourself by making a little “movement club”? How about a group WhatsApp chat where you promise to do a posture routine three times a week and encourage each other if someone falls off the wagon?

Once you get into the habit of regular practice, you will become addicted to how good you feel. As you continue to practise, it will become much easier to find time. Habits generally take one or two months to become engrained. Until then, discipline is your friend. Also, don’t wait for motivation to strike. I think motivation is a bit of a red herring, at least until a habit becomes entrenched. Those of us who practise regularly are not motivated every single day; we stay disciplined and perform the small daily actions that eventually lead to success. Diarize your movement practice and make it as important as anything else you have in your diary.

Second, there are people like me who can help you on an ongoing basis. Find a teacher who resonates with you, who delivers a type of movement you enjoy and, crucially, who offers a type of movement that makes you feel better afterwards. Movement should not make you feel tense, achy or in pain. If it does, your body doesn’t want you to do that type of exercise right now. Movement should make you feel free, loose, balanced and energized afterwards. If staying pain-free long term is your goal, please remember the following three rules.

1. **Quality**: Restore the function of your muscles and the balance of your joints so your body can move more efficiently, with no pain and no tension.
2. **Variety**: Consider if you are moving every part of your body through its full range of motion on a regular basis.
3. **Quantity**: If you follow the first two rules, you will be ready to move a lot more and with more intensity. Too many of us bypass the first two stages and then suffer pain and frustration by doing too much too soon.

Show yourself some love

On a personal level, if you had told me ten years ago that I would not only love to exercise every day, but that my career would be based on movement, I'd have scoffed in your face. Have no illusions about me: I was more inactive than most of my friends and less health-conscious than many of them. Movement changed my life. Things shifted when I began to see movement as a gift, a pleasure and a way to show myself self-compassion. Until that point, I had seen movement as a punishment and I could never get on board with it – so it never stuck.

For many of us, our reluctance to move is caused by a lack of self-compassion: we think we don't deserve to spend time on improving ourselves. We are all worthy. We all deserve to honour and love our body and nourish it in any way we can. You will be a better parent, friend, partner, sibling, employee, employer or child if you are not held back by the physical reality or mental anguish of pain. Movement helps us to become the best version of ourselves and exercising is an essential part of feeling great as a human being.

Find and reclaim your posture power, and you will be rewarded for the rest of your life.

Final posture pointers

1. Rather than thinking too much about how you sit, the angle of your screen, the chair you sit in or your ergonomic desk set-up, think about sitting on a chair and staring at a screen less. If you reduce the amount of time you spend sitting down by even a few minutes a day, this will make a huge difference over the course of your lifetime.
2. Why must we always relax in a chair? Even when we're relaxing and watching TV in the evening, we don't have to sit in a chair. Get on the floor, sit cross-legged, kneel, lie prone, lie supine – do anything that will change your movement profile. Think about hunter-gatherers: lots of relaxing, just not sitting in a chair.

3. At work and at leisure, try and break up your sitting time as much as you can. Not only will this help keep your muscles pumping, but studies show that people who frequently break up their sitting time can have up to 25 per cent less inflammation in their body. Inflammation in the body is associated with a greater risk of most chronic lifestyle diseases.
4. How you spend your leisure time is super important. You may not be able to change how much time you spend sitting down for your job or during your commute, but you *can* change what you do outside of this time. How are you spending your mornings, evenings, lunch breaks, weekends and holidays? How can you squeeze in more movement?
5. Aim to get rid of your pillows. This may take some time for your brain and muscles to adapt, but sleeping without pillows is one of the best things I have done for my posture. Reduce the height of your pillows slowly over time and also work on your posture in other ways. Without pillows, you will be more likely to sleep supine, which is more balanced for the body.
6. Transition to barefoot or minimalistic shoes. This change can take some time (and perhaps a lot of corrective posture exercises to restore lost muscular function), but switching to barefoot or minimalistic shoes is incredibly worthwhile if your goal is to stay pain-free for your whole life. You may want to recruit a movement practitioner to help with the transition. I recommend Vivobarefoot, wildsole, Earth Runners and Feelgrounds for various types of more minimalistic shoes. I ran my half-marathon in wildsole sandals.
7. If you have a child, or plan on having children, allow them to go barefoot for as long as possible. Let them move at their own pace, without support. Wherever possible, keep your children out of seats, highchairs, bouncers, walkers or anything else that props them up before their muscles are ready to hold them up independently.

8. Spend time barefoot outdoors. Some of you may live in a climate where it is warm enough to do this all year round – you have no excuse! If not, do your best, but remember that spending time barefoot outdoors reduces inflammation in your body – due to the principles of "earthing/grounding" – and helps to calm you.
9. Get a squatty potty to change the angle of your pelvis when you go to the loo. Toileting in this new position will not only improve your muscular function but also enable more efficient waste removal.
10. Exercise your eyes. Get outside as often as you can and think about your eye muscles as being part of your posture. Look at things in the near distance, medium distance and far distance. Keep one eye closed and make the other eye do all the work for a bit; swap over. Make your eyes work hard to improve their strength because weak eye muscles will create issues with your eyesight and feed into tension down the spine and shoulders.
11. Invest time in learning to breathe. You could work with a breathwork practitioner (in the case of more serious breathing conditions) or teach yourself via online classes and books. I recommend The Buteyko Method.*
12. In terms of using mouth tape at night, I use MyoTape from Oxygen Advantage. This goes around your mouth, and doesn't force your mouth closed.
13. Get outside more. Just do it, come rain or shine. Being outside is one of the best medicines we have for our mental and physical wellbeing.

* For a list of practitioners, see thebuteykomethod.com

REFERENCES AND FURTHER READING

My website

My YouTube channel

Anthropology and general health

Brogan, K, *A Mind of your Own*, Harper Wave, New York, 2016
Chatterjee, R, *The 4 Pillar Plan*, Penguin Life, London, 2018
Clear, J, *Atomic Habits*, Random House Business, London, 2018
Cregan-Reid, V, *Primate Change*, Octopus Publishing Group, London, 2018
Gokhale, E, *8 Steps to a Pain-Free Back*, Lotus Publishing, Chichester, 2013
Harari, Y N, *Sapiens*, Penguin Random House, London, 2011
Hari, J, *Stolen Focus*, Crown Publishing Group, New York, 2022
Hill, S, *Why the Pill Changes Everything*, Orion Spring, London, 2024
van der Kolk, B, *The Body Keeps the Score*, Penguin Books, London, 2015
Lieberman, D, *Exercised*, Penguin, London, 2021
Lieberman, D, *The Story of the Human Body*, Penguin Books, London, 2013
Maté, G, *When the Body Says No*, Vermilion, 2019
Ober, C, *Earthing*, Basic Health Publications, Laguna Beach, California, 2014

Rutherford, A, *The Book of Humans: The Story of How We Became Us*, Weidenfeld & Nicolson, London, 2018
Shetty, J, *Think Like a Monk*, Thorsons, London, 2020
Walker, M, *Why We Sleep*, Penguin Books, London, 2017
Weaver, L, *Rushing Woman's Syndrome*, Hay House UK, London, 2017

Movement and anatomy

Bowman, K, *Diastasis Recti: The Whole Body Solutions to Abdominal Weakness and Separation*, Propriometrics Press, Carlsborg, Washington, 2016
Bowman, K, *Dynamic Aging*, Propriometrics Press, Carlsborg, Washington, 2017
Bowman, K, *Move Your DNA*, Propriometrics Press, Carlsborg, Washington, 2017
Bowman, K, *Simple Steps to Foot Pain Relief*, BenBella Books, Dallas, Texas, 2016
Bowman, K, *Whole Body Barefoot: Transitioning Well to Minimal Footwear*, Propriometrics Press, Carlsborg, Washington, 2015
Egoscue, P, *The Egoscue Method of Health Through Motion*, New York, Quill, 1992
Egoscue, P, *Pain Free*, Bantam Books, New York, 2021
Hanscom, D, *Back in Control*, Vertus Press, London, 2017
Keil, D, *Functional Anatomy of Yoga*, Lotus Publishing, Chichester, 2017
Myers, T, *Anatomy Trains*, Churchill Livingstone, London, 2013
Riddle, T, *Be More Human*, Penguin Life, London, 2022
Sarno, J, *Healing Back Pain*, Grand Central Life & Style, New York, 2016
Ward, G, *What the Foot?*, Soap Box Books, 2013
Williamson, C, *Muscular Retraining for Pain-Free Living*, Trumpeter Books, Boston, Massachusetts, 2007

Breathwork

McKeown, P, *The Breathing Cure*, OxyAt Books, Dublin, Ireland, 2021
Nestor, J, *Breath*, Penguin Life, London, 2020

Children and parenthood

Armstrong, E, *The Fearless Birth Book*, DK, London, 2024
Hanscom, A, *Balanced and Barefoot*, New Harbinger Publications, Oakland, California, 2016
Reed, R, *Reclaiming Childbirth as a Rite of Passage*, Word Witch Press, Yandina, Queensland, 2021

Studies and other references

Anderson, O, et al., "Bone health in elite Norwegian endurance cyclists and runners: A cross-sectional study", *BMJ Open Sport & Exercise Medicine*, 4(1), 2018

"Baby Carriage", McClung Museum of Natural History & Culture, mcclungmuseum.utk.edu/object-of-the-month/baby-carriage/

Guadalupe-Grau, A, et al., "Exercise and bone mass in adults", *Sports Medicine*, 39(6), 2009, pp.439–468

Mannix, L, "Is good posture overrated?", *The Guardian*, 5 August 2023, theguardian.com/science/2023/aug/06/good-posture-back-pain-how-to-avoid

Morino, S, et al., "Pelvic alignment changes during the perinatal period", *PLoS One*, 14(10), 2019, pmc.ncbi.nlm.nih.gov/articles/PMC6799872/

"Move Your DNA" podcast by Katy Bowman

NHS "Infertility", nhs.uk/conditions/infertility/

Nordstroem, J, "Literature synthesis on neurogenic tremors", Saybrook University, 2021

Obokhare, I, "Fecal impaction: A cause for concern?", *Clinics in Colon and Rectal Surgery*, 25(1), 2012, pmc.ncbi.nlm.nih.gov/articles/PMC3348734/

Popescu, A, "Why staring at screens is making your eyeballs elongate – and how to stop it", *The Guardian*, 14 November 2021, theguardian.com/society/2021/nov/14/eyeballs-screens-vision-nearsightedness-myopia

Satyjeet, F, et al., "Psychological stress as a risk factor for cardiovascular disease: A case-control study", *Cureus*, 12(10), 2020, pmc.ncbi.nlm.nih.gov/articles/PMC7603890/

Shepherd, S, "Why Erling Haaland and Iga Swiatek are taping over their mouths", *The Athletic*, 11 September 2023, nytimes.com/athletic/4844743/2023/09/11/why-sportspeople-taping-over-mouths/

Truslow, W, *Body Poise*, Baltimore, Maryland, The Williams and Wilkins Company, 1943

Uden, H, Scharfbillig, R and Causby, R, "The typically developing paediatric foot: How flat should it be? A systematic review", *Journal of Foot and Ankle Research*, 10(37), 2017, jfootankleres.biomedcentral.com/articles/10.1186/s13047-017-0218-1

Whitcombe, K, Shapiro, L and Lieberman, D, "Fetal load and the evolution of lumbar lordosis in bipedal hominins", *Nature*, 450, 2007, pp.1075–1078

Yosifon, D and Stearns, P N, "The rise and fall of American posture", *The American Historical Review*, 103(4), 1998, pp.1057–1095, doi.org/10.2307/2651198

ENDNOTES

1. Lieberman, D, *The Story of the Human Body*, Penguin Books, London, 2013, pp.180–186
2. Bowman, K, *Move Your DNA*, Propriometrics Press, Carlsborg, Washington, 2017, p.2
3. Lieberman, D, *Exercised*, Penguin, London, 2021, pp.298–336
4. Mannix, L, "Is good posture overrated?", *The Guardian*, 5 August 2023, theguardian.com/science/2023/aug/06/good-posture-back-pain-how-to-avoid
5. Lieberman, D, *Exercised*, Penguin, London, 2021, p.57
6. Ibid, p.56
7. Lieberman, D, *The Story of the Human Body*, Penguin Books, London, 2013, pp.180–186
8. Lieberman, D, *The Story of the Human Body*, Penguin Books, London, 2013, p.19; Cregan-Reid, V, *Primate Change*, Octopus Publishing Group, London, 2018, p.18
9. Lieberman, D, *The Story of the Human Body*, Penguin Books, London, 2013, p.31
10. Cregan-Reid, V, *Primate Change*, Octopus Publishing Group, London, 2018, p.16
11. Lieberman, D, *Exercised*, Penguin, London, 2021, p.17
12. Ibid, p.57
13. Ibid, p.69
14. Ibid, p.55
15. Ibid, p.52
16. Source unknown.
17. Lieberman, D, *Exercised*, Penguin, London, 2021, pp.234–236
18. Ibid, p.237
19 Lieberman, D, *Exercised*, Penguin, London, 2021, p.230
20. Ibid, p.232
21. Ibid, p.125
22. Ibid, p.137
23. Ibid, p.322
24. Ibid, p.56
25. Gokhale, E, *8 Steps to a Pain-Free Back*, Lotus Publishing, Chichester, 2013, p.13
26. Bowman, K, *Move Your DNA*, Propriometrics Press, Carlsborg, Washington, 2017, p.48
27. Ibid, p.32
28. "Baby Carriage", McClung Museum of Natural History & Culture, mcclungmuseum.utk.edu/object-of-the-month/baby-carriage/

29. Lieberman, D, *Exercised*, Penguin, London, 2021, p.187
30. Bowman, K, *Move Your DNA*, Propriometrics Press, Carlsborg, Washington, 2017, p.35
31. Gokhale, E, *8 Steps to a Pain-Free Back*, Lotus Publishing, Chichester, 2013, pp.33, 39, 41
32. Myers, T, *Anatomy Trains*, Churchill Livingstone, London, 2013, pp.198–200
33. Ibid, p.200
34. Lieberman, D, *The Story of the Human Body*, Penguin Books, London, 2013, p.299
35. Yosifon, D and Stearns, P N, "The rise and fall of American posture", *The American Historical Review*, 103(4), 1998, p.1072, doi.org/10.2307/2651198
36. Hari, J, *Stolen Focus*, Crown Publishing Group, New York, 2022, pp.238–244
37. Truslow, W, *Body Poise*, Baltimore, Maryland, The Williams and Wilkins Company, 1943, p.136
38. Lieberman, D, *Exercised*, Penguin, London, 2021, p.21
39. Ibid, p.66
40. Ibid
41. Ibid, pp.119–120
42. Lieberman, D, *Exercised*, Penguin, London, 2021, p.136
43. Ibid, p.216
44. Guadalupe-Grau, A, et al., "Exercise and bone mass in adults", *Sports Medicine*, 39(6), 2009; Anderson, O, et al., "Bone health in elite Norwegian endurance cyclists and runners: A cross-sectional study", *BMJ Open Sport & Exercise Medicine*, 4(1), 2018
45. Lieberman, D, *Exercised*, Penguin, London, 2021, p.131
46. Ibid, p.322
47. Ibid, p.321
48. Cregan-Reid, V, *Primate Change*, Octopus Publishing Group, London, 2018, p.58
49. Lieberman, D, *Exercised*, Penguin, London, 2021, p.105
50. Bowman, K, *Move Your DNA*, Propriometrics Press, Carlsborg, Washington, 2017, p.18
51. Lieberman, D, *Exercised*, Penguin, London, 2021, p.85
52. Ibid, p.54
53. Ober, C, *Earthing*, Basic Health Publications, Laguna Beach, California, 2014, p.23
54. Lieberman, D, *Exercised*, Penguin, London, 2021, p.85
55. Ober, C, *Earthing*, Basic Health Publications, Laguna Beach, California, 2014
56. Ibid, p.9
57. Ibid, p.68
58. Cregan-Reid, V, *Primate Change*, Octopus Publishing Group, London, 2018, p.53

59. Bowman, K, *Move your DNA*, Propriometrics Press, Carlsborg, Washington, 2017, p.159
60. Ibid, p.39
61. Lieberman, D, *Exercised*, Penguin, London, 2021, p.206
62. Cregan-Reid, V, *Primate Change*, Octopus Publishing Group, London, 2018, p.40
63. Ibid, p.48
64. Ibid, p.45
65. Lieberman, D, *Exercised*, Penguin, London, 2021, p.179; Bowman, K, *Move Your DNA*, Propriometrics Press, Carlsborg, Washington, 2017, p.104
66. Lieberman, D, *Exercised*, Penguin, London, 2021, p.214
67. Ibid p.202, 206
68. Ibid, pp.210–211
69. Uden, H, Scharfbillig, R and Causby, R, "The typically developing paediatric foot: How flat should it be? A systematic review", *Journal of Foot and Ankle Research*, 10(37), 2017, jfootankleres.biomedcentral.com/articles/10.1186/s13047-017-0218-1
70. Lieberman, D, *Exercised*, Penguin, London, 2021, p.217
71. Yosifon, D and Stearns, P N, "The rise and fall of American posture", *The American Historical Review*, 103(4), 1998, pp. 1057–1095, doi.org/10.2307/2651198
72. Ibid
73. McKeown, P, *The Breathing Cure*, OxyAt Books, Dublin, Ireland, 2021, p.107
74. Ibid, p.122-140
75. Ibid, p.140
76. McKeown, P, *The Breathing Cure*, OxyAt Books, Dublin, Ireland, 2021
77. Ibid, p.104–105
78. youtube.com/watch?v=cU4ls5ku4Rg
79. McKeown, P, *The Breathing Cure*, OxyAt Books, Dublin, Ireland, 2021, p.100–102
80. Shepherd, S, "Why Erling Haaland and Iga Swiatek are taping over their mouths", *The Athletic*, 11 September 2023, nytimes.com/athletic/4844743/2023/09/11/why-sportspeople-taping-over-mouths/
81. Bowman, K, *Move Your DNA*, Propriometrics Press, Carlsborg, Washington, 2017, p.58
82. Lieberman, D, *Exercised*, Penguin, London, 2021, p.68
83. Ibid, p.308
84. Satyjeet, F, et al., "Psychological stress as a risk factor for cardiovascular disease: A case-control study", *Cureus*, 12(10), 2020, pmc.ncbi.nlm.nih.gov/articles/PMC7603890/
85. Nordstroem, J, "Literature synthesis on neurogenic tremors", Saybrook University, 2021

86. Egoscue, P, *Pain Free*, Bantam Books, New York, 2021
87. Bowman, K, Diastasis Recti: The Whole Body Solutions to Abdominal Weakness and Separation, Propriometrics Press, Carlsborg, Washington, 2016, p.77
88. Bowman, K, Move Your DNA, Propriometrics Press, Carlsborg, Washington, 2017, pp.146–147
89. Obokhare, I, "Fecal impaction: A cause for concern?", Clinics in Colon and Rectal Surgery, 25(1), 2012, pmc.ncbi.nlm.nih.gov/articles/PMC3348734/
90. NHS "Infertility", nhs.uk/conditions/infertility/
91. Morino, S, et al., "Pelvic alignment changes during the perinatal period", PLoS One, 14(10), 2019, pmc.ncbi.nlm.nih.gov/articles/PMC6799872/
92. Ibid
93. Whitcombe, K, Shapiro, L and Lieberman, D, "Fetal load and the evolution of lumbar lordosis in bipedal hominins", Nature, 450, 2007, pp.1075–1078
94. Egoscue, P, The Egoscue Method of Health Through Motion, New York, Quill, 1992, pp.74–75
95. Bowman, K, Move Your DNA, Propriometrics Press, Carlsborg, Washington, 2017, pp.114–115
96. Lieberman, D, Exercised, Penguin, London, 2021, p.66
97. Ibid, p.69
98. Popescu, A, "Why staring at screens is making your eyeballs elongate – and how to stop it", The Guardian, 14 November 2021, theguardian.com/society/2021/nov/14/eyeballs-screens-vision-nearsightedness-myopia

ABOUT THE AUTHOR

Posture Ellie (Eleanor Dalton) is a posture therapist who lives rurally in the beautiful English Peak District National Park with her husband, and fellow posture therapist, Ben. Together they love long countryside walks with Gozo their dog, keeping active and helping people all over the world correct their movement patterns and feel amazing. Future plans involve buying a farm, becoming self-sufficient, hosting retreats and fulfilling a life-long dream of owning a horse (or three).

ACKNOWLEGEMENTS

A really big thank you to everyone who has supported me in some way as I have gone on this journey from being employed, to becoming self-employed, to writing a book! I have already given all my wonderful clients a shout-out (at the very beginning of my book) so will leave this space for more personal acknowledgements.

Firstly, a huge amount of gratitude must be given to my first agent, Edwina (previously of MMB Creative). Thank you so much for reaching out all those years ago and taking a chance on me! Another round of gratitude must be given to my new agent, Sharmaine, the rest of the International Creative Agency team (formerly MMB Creative) and to my publisher, Sophie, and the rest of the Watkins Publishing team. I will be eternally grateful for Watkins for offering me my literary break.

Secondly, to all my friends and family for listening to me endlessly witter on intensely about posture, feet, muscles, barefoot shoes, grounding and the like. I appreciate I am quite annoying and it takes a fair amount of patience to put up with me!

Separate shout-outs must go to my Aunty Helen; for providing sound wisdom and a passionate love for books that rubs off on me. My first 'proper' boss Rollo, the first entrepreneurial character I knew and someone who had a profound effect on me; you showed me a different way of seeing the world and recognising how much potential is in it. To Laura, my first 'proper' yoga teacher, who made me realise that I could leave my job and become self-employed doing something I loved. To my funny, caring sister Antonia for always being there for me when I have one of my many rants or breakdowns and for blessing me with my gorgeous niece and nephew, Sylvie and Rowan.

To my Mum, Anne, for being a reliable and trustworthy parent but, importantly, a true example of an independent woman who showed me what I could achieve if I wanted to. Thank you for never trying to control or steer my ambition (I know you'd have loved it if I'd been more into Maths or Economics, but you had to deal with horses and 'hair-brained schemes') or tell me what to do (except for telling me to hang up wet towels and to stop smearing fake tan everywhere) and for letting me make my own mistakes and giving me the space to figure stuff out for myself. The bar was always set so high by you.

Finally, to my husband, Ben. Running our business and, especially, writing the book, put me 'under the cosh' (see, I do sometimes listen when you rant on about football) and I appreciate your patience, tough love and support. I can't believe I found you, I am so grateful to you and I so look forward to our life together. Thanks for being (wonderfully weird) you.

INDEX

posture ellie